HOW TO
SLEEP
WELL

HOW TO
SLEEP
WELL

Everything You Need to Know about Getting a Good Night's Sleep from Diet, Routine, Environment, Lifestyle, and More

DR. CHRIS IDZIKOWSKI

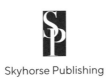

Skyhorse Publishing

First published by Eddison Books Limited

First Skyhorse Publishing Edition 2019

Visit our website at www.skyhorsepublishing.com.

1 3 5 7 9 10 8 6 4 2

Library of Congress Cataloging-in-Publication Data is available on file.

Cover artwork by Steve Rawlings

ISBN: 978-1-5107-4968-9

Printed in Hong Kong
First published in 1999 in the U.S.A. by Penguin Studio Books,
a member of Penguin Putnam Inc., as *The Insomnia Kit*.

ADVICE TO THE READER
This book is not intended as guidance for the treatment of serious health problems; please refer to a medical professional if you are in any doubt about any aspect of your condition.

Contents

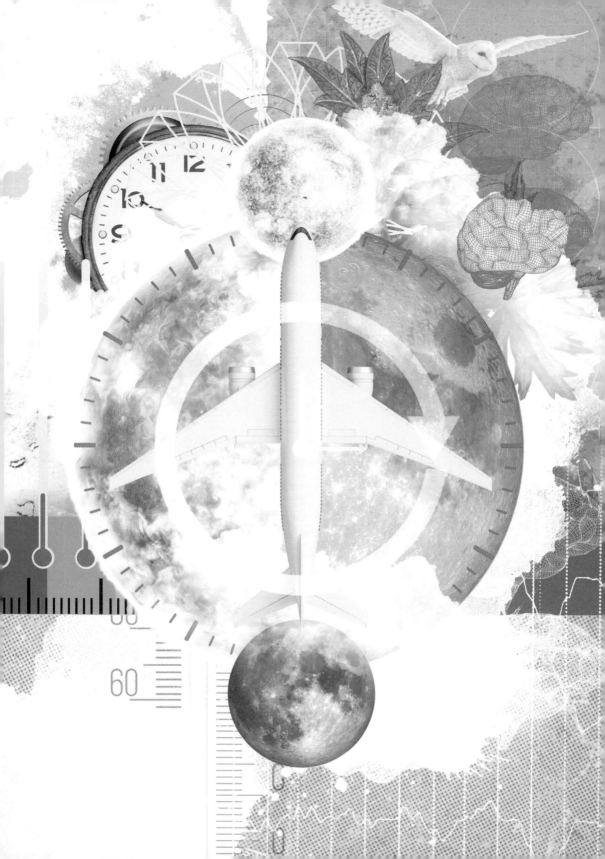

Preface

Sleep has interested me my entire career. It started with one question: How does the brain 'switch off' and 'switch on'? That question immediately led to others: What happens to consciousness when it's fully turned off? What can it do when in this state? The research turned into practical questions of how to help people with sleep disorders before evolving into more research on how sleep disorders affected physical and mental disorders. I did this as a sleep researcher with a background of psychology, psychopharmacology and clinical pharmacology (the latter two involving the investigation of the effects of drugs and medicines on people).

When I started sleep research, sleep medicine was not recognized as a speciality. So to develop the area, I helped set up the British Sleep Society and subsequently the Royal Society of Medicine's (RSM) Sleep Medicine Section. The aim of the former was to provide up-to-date research for those specialities particularly interested in and constantly working in sleep, whereas the latter was aimed at any speciality that needed to keep up to date with what was happening in sleep. One of RSM's strengths is continuous professional development – a place where specialities can meet.

Sleep research in its current form started in the late 1950s to early 1960s with the discovery of REM (dreaming) sleep. The American Academy for Sleep Medicine was founded in 1970 and developed qualifications and careers for American sleep specialists. It is only recently in Europe that a 'somnologist' qualification has been established. Nonetheless, apart from in the United States, there aren't any career routes or formal ways for professionals to qualify as sleep specialists. The technicians, the backbone of any sleep disorders centre, now have a formal system of registration that is recognized internationally (Registered Polysomnographic Technicians – RPSGT).

Sleep continues to fascinate me. It's a time the mind and brain move into such a different state compared to wakefulness. And though I have studied the subject for many years, questions still arise: How does the brain do that? How does the mind follow? Or is it the other way around? Other questions naturally follow. What is to be done if sleep goes wrong? Is it really a problem? The answers to these questions aren't clear-cut, but what I do know is that if you have problems with your sleep, you need to explore them and work out the best solutions for yourself. This book aims to help you in that process so that you are one step closer to a good night's rest.

Introduction

Nearly everyone has lost the ability to sleep at one time or another. Sleep disorders can be devastating. Sleepiness, particularly uncontrolled and unexpected sleepiness, can lead to accidents and poor decisions and sleeplessness can also ruin a person's health and quality of life. This book uses contemporary clinical and research knowledge and it includes my own view of sleep research and sleep medicine, evolved over forty or so years. It examines sleep, disturbed sleep, disordered sleep and sleep disorders. It explains sleep, identifies the problems and suggests remedies. Most of these involve you taking action. Simple over-the-counter panaceas rarely work long-term, so don't expect a 'use this it'll fix it' approach. Sleep isn't like that.

'Sleep rulers', as used in this book, are a subjective measure of your sleep. You describe how you thought you slept, how awake or not you feel, how well you feel, etc. Nowadays there are many devices and apps that claim to measure your sleep. I will mention hardly any in the book for two reasons: 1) many if not all 'claim', albeit honestly, to measure sleep but there are none that I am aware of that actually measure **your** sleep, and **your** wakefulness; 2) I've watched too many companies and websites come and go over the last ten years or so to recommend one, as I can't be sure they'll be in business when the book is published! My favourite device the 'Zeo' was not only a sleep researcher's delight but had all the bells and whistles for supporting cognitive behavioural therapy for insomnia (the 'in' technique) that I could wish for. However, it went bust. Fitness trackers – my favourite became the Jawbone Up3, but that also failed. Both left thousands of users adrift.

So, apart from technology changing, what else has happened in the past twenty years regarding the research of sleep? The science has moved on. There still though, isn't an answer to the basic question: 'What is the function of sleep?' In fact, science has probably created a lot more questions about sleep! Now twenty years' more information, and more and more scientists and clinicians are interested in sleep and we are only a little further forward. What is clear is that:

1. Across species and history sleep adapts to optimize brain and body recovery – sometimes bodily recovery is a by-product of the rest that sleep enforces.
2. Sleep interacts with the body's 24-hour body clock to optimize functioning.
3. The brain probably benefits most from sleep that almost completely disconnects it from both the external world and the body's internal milieu.

I would say the important findings and changes are:

1. The discovery of 'Glymphatics' – part of sleep's function in the brain is to help remove all the metabolic debris that is created while you're awake.
2. The discovery that the ganglion cells in the retina of the eye are particularly blue-light sensitive and feed via exclusive pathways in the optic nerve directly to the brain's 24-hour biological clock. Importantly, and unfortunately, many smartphones, monitors and television sets emit these blue-light frequencies.
3. We've learned that sleep is very different across more mammalian and other species than we've known hitherto. Dolphins can let one brain hemisphere go to sleep while the other remains awake and vice versa. Some seals go one step further and do the same when they are in the sea but allow both hemispheres to work together when they sleep on land!
4. Historically, it was common to have two sleeps in the night, a 'first' sleep, then a period of wakefulness followed by a 'second' sleep. Street lighting put paid to that!
5. Anthropologists have also been at work and found a greater diversity in sleep patterns, where globalization hasn't squashed it.
6. The discovery of orexin (hypocretin), a brain chemical which controls wakefulness (one side of the three-way conductor of sleep: sleep, wake and biological clock).
7. Brain imaging, which has shown that not all of the brain goes to sleep at the same time – not all parts follow the 'sleep' conductor.
8. More sleep disorders centres! This has partly come about from the big increase in the detection of sleep apnoea, the frequency of which may have increased with the increase in the prevalence of obesity.
9. The acceptance of Cognitive Behavioural Therapy for Insomnia (CBT-I) for the treatment of 'insomnia'. Here, the book kind of wins! Many of the techniques employed and suggested in the original are used in CBT-I, it's just that CBT-I has packaged them in a different way, for example, Bootzin Stimulus Control (*see pages 120–22*) or sleep restriction (*see pages 125–26*).
10. And speaking of 'insomnia', the International Classification of Sleep Disorders is now in its third edition and 'insomnia' has for the fourth time been re-defined (*see pages 134–5*)! It has been four times because the original definition by the first sleep disorders research group pre-dated the International Classification.

So, has 'insomnia' actually changed in the past twenty years?

The answer is yes, more or less. Insomnia still is not being able to sleep when you want to but its definition is now qualified with other considerations: is it a clinically significant problem? what has caused it? how long it's lasted for, what it's doing to you and how it can be treated?

The American Academy of Sleep Medicine has led the way in treating sleep disorders for more than two decades. It publishes the International Classification of Sleep Disorders (ICSD), which most sleep experts use as their guide for diagnosis and treatment. There have been a number of changes, probably more than in psychiatric manuals, but importantly, the definition of 'insomnia' has evolved from edition to edition. In the first edition 'insomnia' was defined in terms that were mainly descriptive: 'Sleep onset insomnia', 'Sleep maintenance insomnia' and 'Early morning awakening insomnia'. These descriptions suited the pharmaceutical companies as they helped medical professionals to identify what pills to use (short-acting, long-acting, middle of the night, etc). These treatments were symptomatic, not curative.

An assumption that continued into the second edition of ICSD, was that it was necessary to treat any underlying disorder (such as anxiety) first. However, the second edition began to identify different types of insomnia: psychophysiological (conditioned) insomnia; sleep state misperception; idiopathic insomnia; inadequate sleep hygiene; behavioural insomnia of childhood and insomnia due to either mental disorder or medical disorder, or to drug or substance abuse.

The third edition broke away both from this assumption and the treatment methods. It dropped the sub-types listed on the previous page and came up with: 'Chronic insomnia disorder'; 'Short-term Insomnia disorder' and 'Other insomnia disorder'. Apart from the symptoms, 'chronic' was defined as 'at least three times per week' and 'for at least three months'. It also connected disturbed sleep to daytime dysfunction, e.g. lack of energy, limiting waking activities and fatigue, etc. The full spectrum of insomnia is thought to affect 10 per cent of Western populations, with 30–35 per cent suffering from some of the symptoms.

Short-term insomnia disorder is closer to what I would call sleeplessness as there is usually an identifiable cause. The one-year prevalence among adults is thought to be 15–20 per cent.

Both chronic and short-term insomnia affect more women and the elderly.

In the update it was also suggested that 'insomnia' should be treated in its own right without referring completely to any precipitating disorder. The treatment thus moved from being symptomatic to curative, the main intervention being cognitive behavioural therapy for insomnia (CBT-I). This is a little different to other cognitive treatments as equal emphasis is placed on disruptive and negative thinking with behavioural methods like stimulus control (*see pages 120–22*) and sleep restriction (*see pages 125–26*) as well as sleep education.

I should say that the European Sleep Research Society has also recently published its guidelines on insomnia and its treatment (in 2017). Generally they agree with their American equivalents. Insomnia should not be considered as a consequence of other disorders or simply on its own right but both: as a condition that can develop on its own and in parallel with other disorders. It should always be treated on its own merits. CBT-I is the treatment with the strongest evidence supporting it.

You need to start reading the book to understand how science and the science of sleep have changed, but I will note here how the treatment of insomnia has changed. There are some new medicines whose action I will also explain later (you need to understand the science) but the big advance is the development of CBT-I. This is partly a repackaging of old techniques but it is also coupled with a new understanding of how sleep works. In essence, CBT-I consists of a cognitive part (which teaches you to manage and control your thoughts concerning sleep in a positive and helpful way) and a behavioural part (which enables your body and brain to relearn how to sleep) – and it is all underpinned by you understanding your sleep.

Sleeplessness and insomnia are different though in ordinary usage the meanings are the same. However, for most sleep experts 'sleeplessness' is when you can't sleep but for the most part understand what is preventing sleep from happening. Insomnia, the disorder, is chronically not being able to sleep when you want to and should be able to and the insomnia is causing you distress.

One explanation, which I endorse, is that there are three factors which cause insomnia: predisposition, precipitating and perpetuating. Predisposition refers to both your biological makeup and how your sleep has developed as you've grown. Most, if not all insomniacs, are not born insomniacs (though some parents may disagree!). The precipitating factor is something that causes sleeplessness. This can be anything that causes sleeplessness for a period: having a baby, looking after someone, stress at work, an injury, uncomfortable or dangerous environment, a trauma, difficult commutes, etc. The perpetuating factors are a result of how you cope with the sleeplessness. You may be perpetuating the sleeplessness by managing it in a way that promotes the sleeplessness long after the initial causes have abated. CBT-I aims both to squash those perpetuating factors and enable you to learn to sleep well again.

In this book, first I cover the science of sleep and highlight the changes in the past couple of decades. Then I introduce my 'sleep rulers' so that you can start measuring your sleep. One's memory of sleep is notoriously inaccurate and is often dominated by the previous night, so it is essential to maintain a diary to see how you and other factors are affecting your sleep. Many of the techniques described take time to have an effect. The advantage is that their effects can be enduring. Of course, there are ways to produce instant sleep. You could be knocked on the head with a hammer but you will wake up with a headache! (Of course I know that being knocked on the head does not cause 'sleep' but unconsciousness but hopefully you understand my meaning – and if not, Chapter One should help.)

In the previous edition of this book, I was continually struck by how some things haven't changed. I reported then that 'early in 1998, the US National Sleep Foundation (NSF) conducted a telephone survey of more than a thousand Americans to assess their knowledge about sleep. Many were found to believe risky myths about sleep and 23 per cent acknowledged that they had fallen asleep while driving in the previous year. Some of the myths were:

- The older you get, the fewer hours of sleep you need.
- Raising the volume on the radio will help you stay awake while driving.
- The human body is able to successfully adjust to nightshift work.
- Snoring is not harmful as long as it doesn't disturb the body's need for sleep.'

The 2018 survey contains both good and bad news. On the positive side, it found that of those adults with excellent sleep health, nearly 90 per cent said they felt very effective at getting things done each day, compared to only 46 per cent of those with poor sleep health. On the negative side, the survey found that only 10 per cent of American adults prioritize their sleep over other aspects of daily living, such as fitness, nutrition, work, social life and hobbies and that 59 per cent did consider how much sleep they needed when planning for the next day. The problem with this is that restricted sleep leads to both long-term problems (like poorer mental health) and short-term issues (like being involved in a traffic collision). Madness!

Sleep is both complicated and simple. If you have a problem, the simple part is either to do with your wakefulness or your sleep. Sleeplessness or insomnia are not being able to sleep when you want to and it's reasonable that you should be able to sleep while excessive sleepiness is not being able to stay awake when you should be able to! Both sleeplessness and sleepiness can be quite normal. Life's pressures, stresses and strains all have an impact – so the question is, when has the sleeplessness or sleepiness reached the stage when you need to seek help?

Various parts of this book address these questions. For insomnia to be treated seriously as a condition, you need to have been suffering for at least three nights a week for a period of at least three months. Note the word 'suffering'. This means you have problems both during the night and you feel that it's affecting you during the day. Note also, I don't give a duration and tell you how much sleep you should have, just whether you are suffering. If you pass this threshold you can immediately go to page 76 BUT I would prefer that you do some preliminary reading first (*Chapters One–Four*). Sleepiness is another matter – this time, if you go to page 141 and complete the Epworth Scale and score 10 or more, you should seriously think about going to visit your doctor.

If you're still reading and haven't jumped to another page or chapter, I should say the aim of this book is to put you on the right path for good sleep health and, if you've already gone astray, to try to get you back on track!

Questionnaires and diaries

The first two chapters explain how sleep works and how you can 'measure' your sleep using the sleep-awake ruler. Chapter Three offers advice on how to manage your sleep by taking account of the various factors that affect it and Chapter Four shows you how to cope when sleep needs to fit into the demands of your life.

Chapter Five includes the 20-day sleep diary. I recommend that you fill this in for 10 days, complete the summary and assessments in Chapter Five, and read the advice on dealing with sleep disorders in Chapter Six and then, practicing what you've learned, return to the diary to fill in the remaining 10 days. You will then be able to see if there has been any improvement in your sleep. Chapter Six includes a breathing exercise, a guided visualization and a mantra to aid relaxation and alleviate anxiety and stress, plus a progressive relaxation routine designed to help you go to sleep. Chapter Seven covers major sleep disorders including, among others, specific insomnias, nightmares and sleepwalking, while Chapter Eight outlines some complementary therapies that can help with insomnia or sleep disorders.

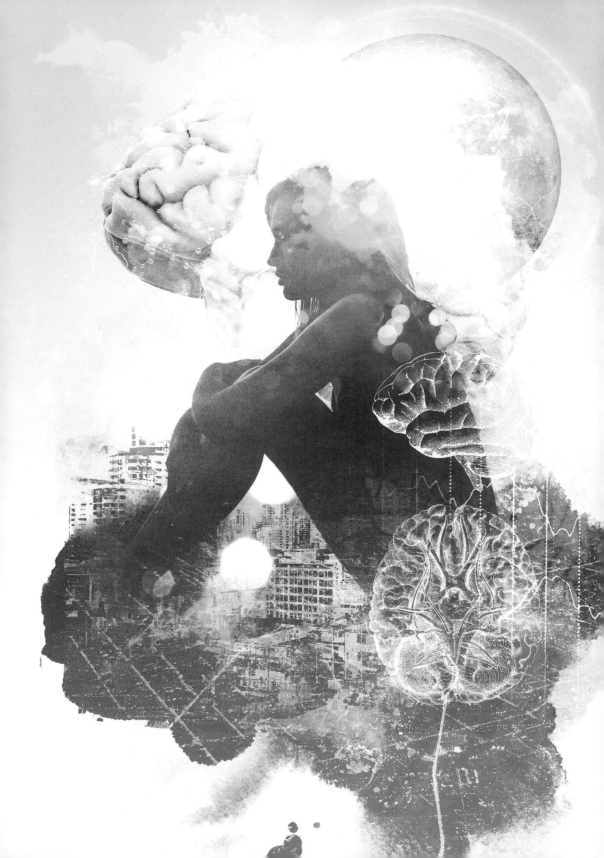

CHAPTER ONE

So you think you're an insomniac?

. . . .

This chapter, and the two following, deal with sleep basics. At the end of them you should have a better idea about the nature of sleep, and how to control it, and also an understanding of whether or not you have a sleep problem.

Over the years there have been many major, international academic surveys measuring the prevalence of insomnia. The range at any one time lies roughly between 10 per cent and 35 per cent of the population, but varies depending on symptoms, how pre-occupied a person is about their symptom, how affected they are during the day, how the country views the symptoms, etc.

Minor problems can turn into long-term problems, so it's worth tackling them quickly. If the princess in the Hans Christian Andersen folk tale really couldn't sleep on top of twenty mattresses and twenty feather beds because there was a pea on the bottom bed, then we need to look at why she became so sensitive in the first place. In the same way, chronic insomniacs may have something in their past that started as a small problem and turned into a big one.

Research has shown that even slight sleep disturbances, so minor that the sleeper does not wake up and is not even aware of any disturbance, will cause daytime performance problems and possibly sleepiness.

From sleeplessness in 1894 to insomnia today

Many people complain that life is tougher, faster and more fraught than it ever used to be, so it is no surprise that people have difficulty sleeping. This may not be correct, as the following quotation from the *British Medical Journal* shows:

> The subject of sleeplessness is once more under public discussion. The hurry and excitement of modern life is quite correctly held to be responsible for much of the insomnia of which we hear: and most of the articles and letters are full of good advice to live more quietly and of platitudes concerning the harmfulness of rush and worry. The pity of it is that so many people are unable to follow this good advice and are obliged to lead a life of anxiety and high tension. Hence the search for some sovereign panacea that will cure the evil. Many are the remedies suggested: hot baths, cold baths, hot drinks, cold drinks, long walks before retiring to rest, and so forth. Different remedies suit different cases ... To be read off to sleep by a gentle voice is, perhaps, the pleasantest way.
>
> 29 September 1894, *British Medical Journal 719*

This was written more than 100 years ago, yet it could have been written today.

In order to understand sleep problems it is useful to understand how sleep relates to physiology. In many countries, the primary treatment of insomnia by the medical profession is through the prescription of sleeping pills (also known as hypnotics). Many people also try to treat themselves by using alcohol or over-the-counter sleep preparations. But using a medicine just to treat a symptom is like using a hammer to fix a TV set. If you are lucky it may work the first time, but next time you might break the TV!

Brain and mind

We do not understand much about the mind or the brain, but I will put forward my own particular views, based on more than forty years of research in the area, so that you can start to get to grips with how your sleep is affected by both biological and mental events. I am going to leave out theorists and practitioners such as Freud because there is not enough space in this book to examine their ideas, but we need to do some work on the brain and the mind. There now follows the shortest course in neuroscience and philosophy that you are ever likely to come across.

Brain

The end of the nineteenth century and the beginning of the twentieth saw a lot of progress in the field of neurology, the medical science that deals with problems associated with the nervous system. It became apparent that there were centres in the brain containing orexin, a neuropeptide (one type of brain chemical messenger) that controlled wakefulness. If those centres were not active then a person would become unresponsive (although not necessarily asleep).

Sleeping sickness, otherwise known as epidemic lethargic encephalitis, provided many of the clues. It not only causes extreme sleepiness but also, at other times, extreme sleeplessness. It can switch around the usual light–dark, activity–rest pattern. Patients remain awake during the night and asleep during the day. The condition was not investigated thoroughly until a major epidemic during the First World War when the Austrian neurologist Von Economo (who discovered the disease) described the specific brain centres that were involved with the control of wakefulness and sleep.

The 1990s film *Awakenings*, starring Robert de Niro and Robin Williams, has increased awareness of epidemic lethargic encephalitis. It describes the use of the medicine L-dopa in the 'awakening' of a number of patients who had remained trapped in a rigid and inarticulate state for many years. L-dopa is a substance that occurs naturally in the body – it is one of the neurotransmitters (another type of brain chemical messenger) that control the awake and sleep states.

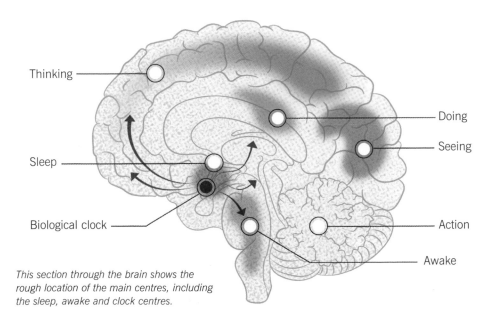

Thinking

Doing

Seeing

Sleep

Biological clock

Action

Awake

This section through the brain shows the rough location of the main centres, including the sleep, awake and clock centres.

This shows how the sleep, awake and clock systems interact when you are awake. For normal sleep to take place, the sleep system needs to be active and the awake system switched off.

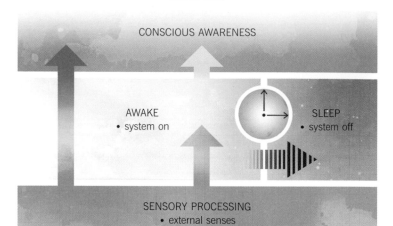

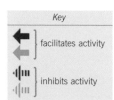

The main point is that sleep is an active brain state and that without specific sleep centres working properly and wake centres able to shut down, sleep cannot take place. The diagram above shows how these systems might interact. It also shows a 'clock'. The clock is connected to the awake system – as well as the sleep system. This biological clock (named the suprachiasmatic nucleus) although small, has a huge number of connections throughout the brain, some of which connect to the sleep systems.

Shown on page 17 is a slice through the human brain, indicating the rough locations of the main 'centres'. The 'clock' centre is located in the hypothalamus, which is also involved in the regulation of eating, drinking and sex. The 'sleep' centre is located in a region that is also involved with the control of body temperature. The regions involved in the control of sleep, awake and clock are not located in areas that are easy to control by voluntary methods. Animals with electrodes implanted in the right parts of the brain can be trained to sleep on command by using conditioning techniques, but this is not a technique that can readily be used on people!

Mind

Sleep is a state that can be recognized in many animals, but in man it is nevertheless a state of mind, or non-mind. The sleep-awake and clock centres interact with higher centres in the brain and inevitably must interact with the mind.

Most neuroscientists argue that the pattern of nerve cell (neuron) firing produces a mental state. Estimates for the number of neurons in the human brain have ranged from

10 billion to 1 trillion. Recent work estimates that out of about 85 billion, 12–15 billion are involved with those areas of the brain that deal with higher functions such as thinking and personality; 70 billion with control of movement and musculature and about 1 billion are in the brainstem and spinal neurons. The brainstem is the lower part of the brain that connects the spinal cord with the brain. This is also the area that contains parts of the 'awake' centre. Even if you consider only the raw numbers, without considering the connections between the neurons, and the fact that neurons have more than one connection (some may have thousands), then you can imagine that even with current technology we are nowhere near to achieving a simulation of any mental state on a computer.

The suprachiasmatic nucleus (biological clock) consists of only 40–80,000 neurons, yet its effects can be very powerful. For some people, jet lag is their first experience of not being able to control sleep on demand (it never was on demand, but their sleep could mould itself to their lifestyle) and the biological clock is a major factor in causing this. Mind and consciousness are inseparable, but curiously, though mind may go to sleep, it is still rare to see any discussion concerning sleep in contemporary debates on mind and consciousness.

The table shown below outlines possible levels of consciousness and also serves as a reminder of various common waking experiences that are not simply involved with thinking. Autonomic systems, that control functions such as heart rate, basic breathing and sweating do not appear to sleep. Many reflexes such as the knee-jerk are inhibited during sleep. General reactivity goes down. This varies depending on the stage of sleep (*see page 31*).

Sleepy awareness refers to that twilight time when someone is not yet fully asleep and still has some idea what is going on around them. Automatic skills refer to highly learned simple movements that do not demand attention – for example, turning the pillow over.

Levels of consciousness	Waking experiences
Conscious self-awareness	Deliberate inner speech
Conscious awareness	Deliberate recall
Alert awareness	Recalled mental images
Asleep	Driving without attention
Sleepy awareness	Daydreaming
Automatic skills	Inattention
Reactivity	Reality aware
Reflex	Inner voice or someone else's?
Autonomic	Environment or location aware

Alert awareness, conscious awareness and conscious self-awareness are in the domain of consciousness. To distinguish man from animals, debates take place as to whether animals are aware of themselves. Sleep clearly affects the higher levels shown in the table and to a lesser extent the lower levels. This does not necessarily mean that processing to support the higher levels stops during sleep; it might just be the awareness of self-processing.

Most sleep research does not deal with consciousness, certainly not with this level of detail. This is partly because it is not possible to ask many of these questions in laboratory experiments and with animals it is difficult, although not impossible, to define the level of consciousness. It is possible to ask questions dealing with alertness, and the ability to respond, and to quantify the changes.

Brain, mind and sleep

The main points we have covered above are that sleep depends on both brain and mind. If the sleep, awake or clock centres are biologically damaged (by using common drugs such as caffeine or alcohol, or drugs of abuse, or by strokes, injury, age and so on) then sleep will be disturbed. Equally, sleep will not come if the mind is upset. Disturbed sleep can be either neuronic (based on neurons) or neurotic (based on mental state). Neuronic theories include all hormonal and other biological influences on sleep. In 1895, one of the ideas circulating among physiologists was that the neurons shrank during sleep. The idea was that shrinkage broke the connecting pathways between neurons and sleep ensued. Neurotic theories do not imply mental disorder, they just define the mental structures involved in sleep. Dr Phil Barnard (formerly Medical Research Council, UK) suggests that sleep is a state when 'self' moves into a state of existential safety by suspension of focal awareness. This is achieved when a number of mental variables – body status, safety, control, self-status and goal-status – reach a specific threshold.

Unfortunately, the important neural or mental components cannot be measured easily. So this book approaches the problem of sleep disorder by measuring and describing objective and subjective sleep and by examining all the variables that we know affect sleep. The sleep-awake-clock model is then used to describe what may be going wrong and how to remedy the problem or problems.

What is sleep?

Sleep is usually defined as a time when an animal stops responding to its surroundings. Most animals close their eyes. Many adopt a specific posture – dogs and cats curl up, bats hang upside down. To distinguish sleep from coma and death, scientists note that this state is reversible!

With human beings, we are used to thinking of sleep as a time when we stop, more or less completely, being aware of anything. For some, it can be a sanctuary, a place to escape. For others, such as sleep apnoeics (*see page 139*) it is a nuisance, often making them drop off unexpectedly during the day. In others still, the boundaries between sleep and waking can be blurred.

What is normal sleep?

There is no straightforward answer to this question, as sleep varies so much, with age, between individuals and with circumstance that it is difficult to give a precise answer. The time a person sleeps, the duration of the sleep, the continuity of the sleep and the recuperative value of the sleep is an amalgamation of various factors, including general health, habits and family demands (*see page 24*). Normality needs biological, personal and social frames of reference before an answer can be given. If you feel that there is something wrong with your sleep, and you do not feel well or cannot cope, and if the problem has been going on for several months, then read on.

When to sleep

In industrialized societies sleep is a compromise between biology and the demands of society – it is said that Thomas Edison created havoc by inventing the electric light bulb. There is evidence to suggest that normal sleep does not consist of one block of 7½ hours during the night. It is more likely that our biology is designed to allow us to sleep for about 6 hours during the night and 1½ hours during the day. The cultures where this pattern of sleep can be seen – the siesta cultures – have virtually disappeared (*see page 42*). Sleeping just once in 24 hours is called monophasic sleep, whereas broken sleep is polyphasic. In evolutionary terms, polyphasic animals are the most common, whereas monophasic animals have evolved more recently. Polyphasic patterns of sleep are the most common.

Nocturnal animals are generally active during the night but get some sleep; they sleep during the day but are also active. Diurnal (daytime) animals are more active during the day but also get lots of naps, and vice versa during the night. How well an animal can manage in its environment depends largely on the sense organs it uses. Animals that rely largely on the visual system are likely to be diurnal and will get most of their sleep during the night. Other influences such as satiety (how well-fed the animal feels), body and brain temperature, the previous duration of wakefulness and safe location all contribute to the likelihood of going to sleep.

As societies have become more information-sensitive, the need to maintain high levels of awareness has gone up. Sleep obviously reduces awareness, but even naps are associated with periods of poor information processing. The constant demand for alertness during the day not only prevents daytime sleep, but also has an impact on night-time sleep. However, you only need to look at pre-school children, people on holiday and the retired to see sleep reappearing during the day.

One piece of advice given in many magazine articles is not to nap during the day. I will return to this later (*see pages 55, 60 and 64–6*) but it is worth noting that this is not necessarily good advice: it very much depends on the circumstances. Any sleep, however short, will reduce the pressure to sleep. In an ideal biological world, napping (polyphasic) sleep might be best, as the body is never unduly stressed. This contrasts with monophasic sleep patterns where pressure builds to a maximum during wakefulness and this sleep pressure is then reduced during sleep.

If an elderly person prefers to have a long daytime nap, and accepts that this means less sleep during the night, then that is fine (sorry, carers!). It is the amount of sleep over a 24-hour period that is important, rather than the amount of sleep that takes place during the night.

How long should I sleep?

Again, this is a common question. There is no straightforward answer because so many different factors need to be considered. However, you can say that good sleepers fall asleep quickly and have serene, deep and uninterrupted sleep; they do not snore; they wake up feeling refreshed and do not feel sleepy during the day; they feel that their sleep is enough (whatever it is).

Some people are constitutionally short sleepers (around $4\frac{1}{2}$ hours) but they do not usually complain about their short sleep if they feel well and are not sleepy or tired during the day. They may be worried about sleeping so little, but there is no need to if they feel OK and are satisfied with the way they are functioning. If they are happy with their lives, then the short sleep is a benefit, not a problem. They are probably happy because they are doing something productive and have the edge on everyone else! It is very difficult to turn yourself into a short sleeper if your genetic makeup hasn't made you one.

By contrast, poor sleepers may snore and wake up more than once during the night. They may feel tired and sleepy and drop off to sleep during the day; or they may feel tired but not be able to sleep during the day, as well as feeling irritable and miserable. You know if you are a poor sleeper.

In the 1950s the American Cancer Society conducted a survey to try to identify factors involved in the development of cancers. This included a question about sleep duration. They found that the majority slept approximately 7½ hours, give or take 1½ hours. So, most of the population slept between 6 and 9 hours.

A small reduction in total sleep may not matter too much, as the lighter stages of sleep tend to be lost if the amount of time allowed for sleep is habitually reduced. In adults, nearly half of sleep consists of light sleep, a quarter of deep sleep and another quarter of REM (rapid eye movement, or dreaming) sleep. If you lose sleep one night, then the proportion of deep sleep and REM sleep increases the following night. Any deficit can be made up at weekends.

One study looked at nuns in a convent whose lifestyle forced them to have less sleep than the average. The nuns were given a dispensation to take part in the study, which allowed them to sleep as long as they liked in the morning. Their sleep rapidly moved back to the average, suggesting that even after years of training, it was impossible to learn to sleep less.

Prospective studies conducted indicate that there is a health risk for adults under 65 if sleep is less than 6 hours or more than 8 hours. Adults over 65 don't risk anything with long or short sleep (within reason).

Long sleepers also feel that they have a problem, or in the case of adolescents, parents may feel that they have a problem. Sleep of 10 hours or more is unusual, but not something to worry about. Greater than this, or if it has changed suddenly, then it is useful to examine what is causing the extra sleep. If the sleepiness intrudes into the day then it should certainly be examined, as it may be pointing to disorders that are disturbing sleep during the night (*see Chapter Seven*).

How long should it take me to fall asleep?

The time taken to go to sleep is normally between 5 and 20 minutes. If it takes longer than 30 minutes, then people start to wonder what has gone wrong.

How long should it take me to wake up?

For most people, waking up is not an issue – the alarm clock goes off, and even if they feel (and look) like zombies, they get up and go. Experimental studies have shown though that it takes around 20 minutes to shake off sleep in the morning. This is called sleep inertia and performance is affected during this time. If you always find it difficult to wake up and you find that you always have difficulty going to bed and getting to sleep, then you might be suffering from a biological clock disorder called delayed-sleep-phase syndrome (*see page 145*).

How often should I dream?

Provided the dreams are not nightmares and are not leaving you drained, the maximum a person can dream depends on the amount of time spent in REM sleep (*see page 32*). The ultradian cycle determines the timing of the dreams, which could be expected every 90 minutes. What is not clear is who recalls their dreams. If a person is woken up in a sleep laboratory or a sleep disorders centre in the REM stage and asked what is going on in his or her mind, the sleeper is invariably dreaming. Awareness probably continues beyond the point marked under asleep in the table on page 19 so how lightly you sleep is important. Also, the length of time between a dream finishing and waking up will contribute to the chances of recalling a dream.

Factors affecting sleep

Heredity has a major effect on sleep depth and duration. Learned factors include what your parents (grandparents, nanny or babysitter) did to you when you were a baby and a youngster and what habits you have picked up over the years. In addition, environmental factors (such as bed, bedroom, latitude, season) and personal factors (such as good or poor health, menstrual cycle, menopause, age and so on) contribute to your sleep. (*See diagram opposite.*)

Sleep rulers

A vital feature of this book is the use of the sleep-awake ruler, which will be explained in detail in the next chapter. Using it is the first step to logging what you are doing and what your sleep is doing. Most changes in sleep take time. Some of the changes can be progressive, like those associated with growing old. Others can be faster, changes within the seasons, the month, a week or days. Some of the changes occur within one night. In order to understand and appreciate these changes yourself, you need to measure what is happening. Your memory is not good enough. Sleep affects memory, so you need to write down what is happening to you in some form of diary. The sleep-awake ruler is one way of doing this. (A 20-day blank diary with rulers is provided in Chapter Five.)

Factors affecting sleep

Inherited factors
- Long versus short sleepers
- Depth of sleep

Learned factors
- Bed habits
- Sleeping habits

Family
- Bed-partner
- Children
- Family members

Habits
- Diet
- Drugs
- Exercise
- Smoking
- Alcohol
- Caffeine
- Bed-time routines

Personal health
- Hormonal status
- Age
- Weight
- Illness
- Medical history

Social
- Work
- Shiftwork
- Peer demand

Early learning
- Time to bed
- Continuity
- Wake-up time
- Sleep position
- Awoken by environmental factors
- Association of melatonin with sleep
- Sharing bed/sleeping alone

Environmental factors
- Latitude
- Bedroom factors
- Temperature
- Humidity
- Noise
- Bed surface

A wide variety of factors can affect your sleep – some of which you may not even be aware of.

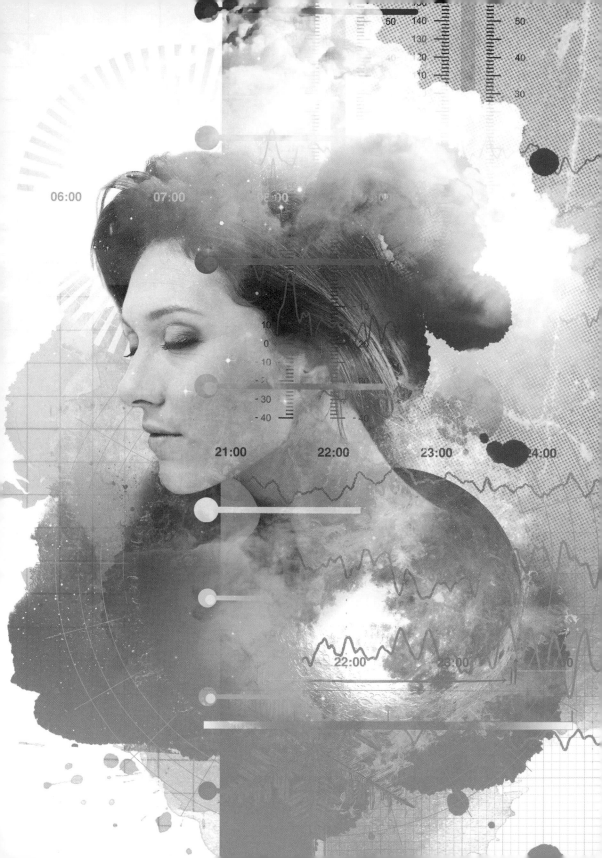

CHAPTER TWO

How to measure sleep

· ·

Over the years I have measured sleep in various ways, using electroencephalography (EEG machines which measure brain activity using electrodes glued to the scalp) in laboratory settings, portable EEGs, actigraphy, various questionnaires and subjective ratings scales. For about a quarter of a century I have been using a particular form of sleep log, which I have called the sleep-awake ruler. It allows patients a convenient, fast and intuitive way to describe what has happened to them during the night.

The sleep-awake ruler

The ruler is divided up into two 12-hour lengths. This is because displaying 24 hours on one ruler on one piece of paper is difficult and the print may be too small for an elderly person to read. One ruler is for measuring, recording and displaying sleep during the night and the other one is for the day (*see below*). The rulers are based on the 24-hour clock, so 1:00 pm becomes 13:00, 10:00 pm becomes 22:00 and so on.

The night ruler starts at 21:00 and finishes at 09:00, while the day ruler starts at 09:00 and finishes at 21:00. In order to record significant sleep events we need to use some symbols. These are shown in the sleep key on the page opposite.

The first ruler (*see page 29*) shows what could be described as a normal night's sleep. The sleeper goes to bed around 22:45 and within a few minutes tries to go to sleep; falls asleep quickly, again within a few minutes; sleeps for around 7½ hours; wakes up, stays in bed for a few minutes, decides not to return to sleep and gets up.

The second ruler (*see page 29*) also shows a completed sleep ruler, but for someone who is having great difficulties with sleep. The sleeper goes to bed about 22:00, but does not try to sleep until 23:00. They then take nearly an hour to fall asleep, but wake up again after about 1½ hours. Half an hour later, they manage to get back to sleep, but it is a restless and disturbed sleep. Eventually, the sleeper settles down, but wakes up

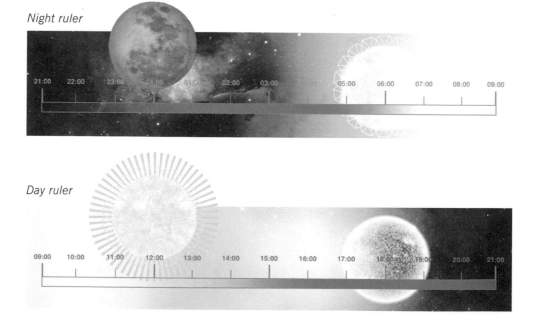

Night ruler

21:00 22:00 23:00 24:00 01:00 02:00 03:00 04:00 05:00 06:00 07:00 08:00 09:00

Day ruler

09:00 10:00 11:00 12:00 13:00 14:00 15:00 16:00 17:00 18:00 19:00 20:00 21:00

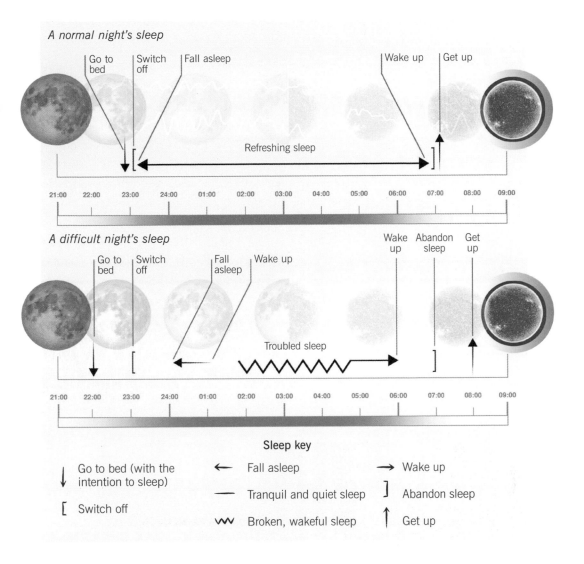

A normal night's sleep

Go to bed | Switch off | Fall asleep | Wake up | Get up

Refreshing sleep

21:00 22:00 23:00 24:00 01:00 02:00 03:00 04:00 05:00 06:00 07:00 08:00 09:00

A difficult night's sleep

Go to bed | Switch off | Fall asleep | Wake up | Wake up | Abandon sleep | Get up

Troubled sleep

21:00 22:00 23:00 24:00 01:00 02:00 03:00 04:00 05:00 06:00 07:00 08:00 09:00

Sleep key

↓ Go to bed (with the intention to sleep)

[Switch off

← Fall asleep

— Tranquil and quiet sleep

⌄⌄⌄ Broken, wakeful sleep

→ Wake up

] Abandon sleep

↑ Get up

earlier than they had hoped. They stay in bed for another hour before giving up trying to sleep, but remain in bed anyway before getting up an hour later. By the end of this book, you will understand many of the reasons why this person's sleep is so disturbed.

Finally, the sleep rulers need to have additional notes to try to assess what factors are disturbing sleep. A few are listed on the next page. A more comprehensive list and discussion are found in the diary section (*see pages 76–8*).

Now that the rulers have been introduced, they can be used to increase the precision of my description of sleep-awake mechanisms. The sleep onset diagram

COMMON SLEEP DISTURBERS

- children
- dreaming
- toilet
- snoring partners
- restless partners

- partners who have other ideas than sleep
- room temperature
- uncomfortable bed/ bedclothes

- noisy pets
- thinking
- worries

(*see below*) shows what happens to someone who takes a while to go to sleep. The sleeper goes to bed at a time when the awake system is beginning to run down. As the evening progresses, most people start routines that begin to relax and prepare them for the night's sleep. Coupled with this, and the connection is not clear, circadian clock activity (*see page 33*) is also optimized to allow sleep to take place. An index of this is core body temperature. It has been found that most people go to sleep in the evening when this is decreasing (it usually peaks in the early evening). Core temperature runs on a 24-hour cycle, with the peak occurring early evening and the trough taking place early morning around dawn.

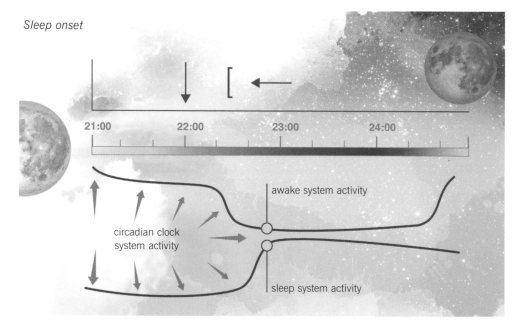

Sleep onset

21:00   22:00   23:00   24:00

awake system activity

circadian clock system activity

sleep system activity

This person goes to bed as their awake system begins to wind down. As this happens, the activity of the circadian (biological) clock allows sleep to take place and the sleep system then begins to take over.

There is more happening than is shown in the sleep onset illustration. In the hours of darkness, melatonin is secreted from the pineal gland. Many other hormones secrete more or less during or prior to sleep – prolactin, testosterone and thyroid-stimulating hormones. In fact, so many of the body's physiological systems are changing, it is surprising how many people can fall asleep quickly and easily!

If you have not already started to wonder at how complicated sleep seems to be, it doesn't get any easier once you are asleep! Sleep is not continuous. You do not simply switch off, stay switched off and then wake up. In adults, a 90-minute rhythm punctuates sleep. This rhythm seems to be dependent on brain size. Animals with small brains have a faster rhythm – for example, mice at about 15 minutes; whereas animals with large brains have a slower rhythm (elephants at 100 minutes). Babies' rhythm is around 60 minutes and as the brain matures and enlarges the rhythm slows to the adult 90 minutes. This rhythm is called ultradian rhythm because it is shorter than the 24-hour circadian rhythm.

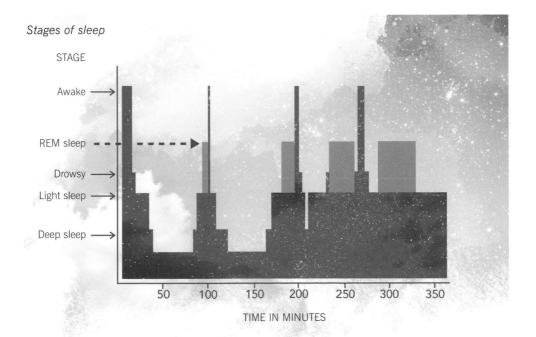

Stages of sleep

There are five sleep stages as shown above. The graph shows the average duration of each stage for a youngish adult.

Ultradian rhythm

This is an important rhythm for those with sleep problems, because it punctuates sleep with wakefulness. It is known as the REM–REM cycle ultradian rhythm, because it is usually measured by determining the time from the onset of one bout of REM to the next. REM, or dreaming, does not just occur at the end of the night, but repeats itself. Usually, the first REM period is quite short (10–15 minutes) and it progressively lengthens during the night, so that it is more than 45 minutes by the end.

As sleep changes from light sleep to REM sleep, there can be periods of wakefulness. The diagram below uses the sleep ruler to illustrate someone who is continuously asleep for 7 hours, without apparent interruption. But the EEG would show interruptions to sleep. There might even be EEG wakefulness, but not long enough either for the sleeper to recall it, or for the sleep to be sufficiently impaired to result in daytime sleepiness. As you get older, the interruption becomes longer and you may become aware that you are awake. If there are problems that you are worried about and you start thinking about them, this may disrupt your sleep enough to prevent you returning to sleep. For the elderly, the circadian cycle is weaker and medical conditions may also lighten sleep, so that these normal interruptions have an even greater impact on sleep.

The function of this rhythm is completely unknown. When it was first noted in the early days of sleep research, the suggestion was that mammals needed to awaken occasionally to check their surroundings for predators. In the 1930s, Nathaniel Kleitman, one of the most eminent researchers into sleep, advocated the existence of a basic

REM–REM cycle and wakefulness in normal sleepers

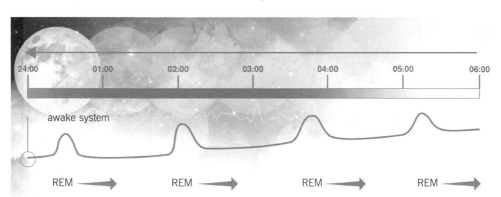

The REM–REM cycle continues throughout sleep, each period of REM becoming progressively longer. The changeover from light sleep to REM sleep may cause wakefulness – even though the sleeper may not realize it.

rest-activity cycle. All known terrestrial animals, not just mammals, have a rest-activity cycle. There are various rhythms in adults that run on a cycle of roughly 70–90-minutes: these include respiration and digestive tract motility (*see page 36*). There is some evidence that these rhythms also affect other mental functions. Snacking behaviour, for example, runs on a 90-minute cycle.

Circadian cycles

There are numerous 24-hour rhythms that are controlled by the circadian or biological clock, including the body temperature curve. Peak temperature occurs early in the evening. Generally, you fall asleep more easily when body temperature starts to go down. Lowest body temperature occurs in the early hours of the morning (around 04:00 for many people) and this is the time when it is easiest to fall asleep. Body temperature then rises until awakening. The body temperature rhythm and other cycles controlled by the biological clock are difficult, if not impossible, to control voluntarily. Difficulties with jet lag and shiftwork are caused by the clock running at an inappropriate time, causing difficulties in sleeping. Growth hormone has a 24-hour cycle that is strongly related to deep sleep, so peak secretion takes place early in the morning (*see below*).

Circadian curves

The biological clock controls the rhythms of body temperature and growth hormone, both of which are related to sleep.

• • • • • body temperature
━━━ growth hormone

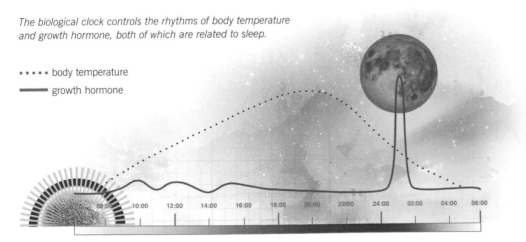

Sleep dynamics

When sleep is investigated using EEG, it is striking how dynamic a process it is. The brain does not simply switch off and lie dormant. It still reacts to the environment and the internal state of the body and it also monitors sleep itself. If someone's sleep is disrupted, then various mechanisms come into play to try to compensate for the disturbance. Brain imaging has shown that not all the brain falls asleep at the same time.

Sleep rebound

If someone is sleep-deprived, then the pressure for sleep increases. Normally, a healthy adult's sleep consists of roughly 25 per cent deep sleep (slow-wave sleep), 25 per cent REM sleep and 50 per cent light sleep (stage 2). If you normally sleep for 8 hours a night, that would be 2 hours deep sleep and 2 hours REM sleep. If you are prevented from sleeping for 2 nights, do you require 24 hours continuous sleep to recover? Experience tells us this does not usually happen without the intervention of drugs or illness. Usually, deep sleep takes priority, followed by REM sleep. The first night is not completely taken up by the 4 hours of deep sleep that is missing (that would be 6 hours deep sleep altogether), but it does take up a substantial amount of that time. The rest of the first recovery night is primarily REM sleep. The second recovery night mops up most of the remaining deep sleep and a lot of REM sleep is also recovered. As REM sleep is associated with dreaming, that can mean that some people experience a lot of dreaming. Sleep rebound leads to the compensatory increase in these stages on recovery nights. The only casualty is light sleep. This virtually disappears in the recovery nights and is lost. Initially, light sleep was regarded as a 'filler' stage, but it seems it may have other roles – for instance, it may be important for some kinds of memory.

REM pressure

By using an EEG machine it is theoretically possible to deprive people of particular stages of sleep. In practice it is difficult because of the compensatory systems in the brain. REM sleep deprivation involves waking someone up whenever he or she goes into REM. In the first cycle of sleep this is quite easy as it is of fairly short duration (about 10–15 minutes). The second cycle normally consists of more REM sleep and again, this is relatively easy to disrupt. It is much more difficult in the third cycle as the brain is already trying to compensate for the REM that has been lost in the first two cycles. The ultradian rhythm is disturbed and REM starts sooner. If this REM is disrupted, then the fourth cycle REM starts sooner still and similarly, the fifth. By the second night of deprivation there is a lot of REM trying to get in, so the night generally becomes very

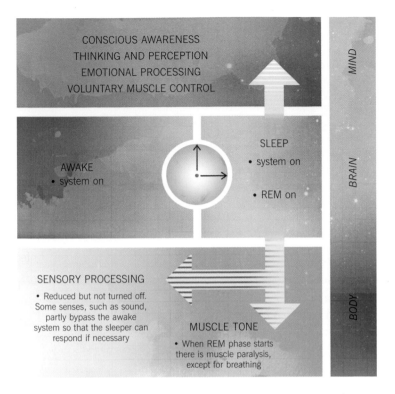

CONSCIOUS AWARENESS
THINKING AND PERCEPTION
EMOTIONAL PROCESSING
VOLUNTARY MUSCLE CONTROL

MIND

AWAKE
• system on

SLEEP
• system on

BRAIN

• REM on

SENSORY PROCESSING
• Reduced but not turned off.
Some senses, such as sound,
partly bypass the awake
system so that the sleeper can
respond if necessary

BODY

MUSCLE TONE
• When REM phase starts
there is muscle paralysis,
except for breathing

When the sleep system is active, conscious awareness is inhibited, thus allowing the awake system to remain off. Muscle paralysis is induced as each REM phase begins, intensifying the general muscle relaxation that has already occurred during other sleep stages.

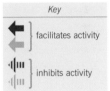

Key

facilitates activity

inhibits activity

disrupted. This demand for REM is known as REM pressure.

There is a similar and stronger demand for deep sleep. In fact, to deprive a person of deep sleep soon means total deprivation, because the demand for deep sleep becomes so intense that the subject has to be continually woken up to prevent him or her from going into deep sleep.

A simple model of sleep

When I come to sleep problems later on in the book, I will be elaborating on what is basically a simple model of sleep, illustrated above. There is a division between mental and biological mechanisms, with only emotions cutting across boundaries. This model is there to act as a temporary summary. The bottom of the diagram shows that, during REM sleep, when the sleep system is switched on and when the REM phase of sleep has started, there is an active paralysis of the body muscles (except for breathing). So the general muscle relaxation that takes place (in people without sleep problems) when sleep begins and in the non-REM stages of sleep is further intensified by an active mechanism that induces paralysis. This active state of paralysis is one of the parts that can go wrong in various sleep disorders, such as narcolepsy (*see pages 137–39*) and REM behaviour disorder (*see page 150*). Most people have suffered from sleep paralysis – waking up and finding that they can't move for 10–30 seconds (*see page 149*). It can be a frightening experience, but it simply means that the brain hasn't woken up yet! It occurs more often in people suffering from jet lag or doing shiftwork and for some genetic reason, the Japanese seem to suffer more from this than Westerners.

Sleep and other bodily and mental functions

It is not surprising that sleep is associated with changes in many mental and bodily functions. A state that occupies about a third of everyone's lives is bound to have an impact. For example, sleep affects both the senses and the memory. Sleep dampens the sensitivity of the senses, but seems to improve memory by strengthening memory traces. The former effect promotes sleep, whereas the latter improves daytime memory function.

Breathing becomes more shallow during sleep, but in snoring and sleep apnoea (stopping breath) breathing is so impaired that sleep becomes disturbed, which can result in sleepiness, tiredness, fatigue, poor concentration, appetite for food, increased blood pressure, involvement in road traffic accidents, etc. The 90-minute sleep cycle rhythm (*see page 31*) can also be found in the digestive system, but only in fasting conditions. Again, the relationship exists, although the functional importance of it is not clear.

Development of human sleep

The box on the page opposite illustrates in a general way how an individual's sleep develops. In babies, the ultradian rhythm, running at around 60 minutes, is much shorter than in an adult. Their sleep is also much more distributed throughout the day in early life, but as the months and years go by, the sleep is consolidated into the night. Melatonin secretion from the pineal gland reaches a peak at the end of the first year of life. The process of sleep is not rigid and unchangeable. The brain systems involved provide a foundation, but learning also contributes to how sleep develops. Mental states, intimately related to the brain, clearly exert an impact as well. An adult's sleep is a fusion of a large number of different actors – so many that it is surprising that more people don't suffer from sleep problems. There is little agreement on what the function of sleep is, but this may be because the question is not particularly clear. What is the

SLEEP DEVELOPMENT
Human sleep begins with sleep during the day and the night.

↓

A process of learning, conditioning and training associates night-time with continuous
sleep and daytime with continuous wakefulness.

function of wakefulness? There are many possible answers for both states. To make
matters worse, much of the research so far has concentrated on Western industrialized
man, so much of the speculation has been extremely focused. Nevertheless, sleep
appears to be a vital state – animal experiments and neurological disorders that produce
total insomnia both show this. Total loss of sleep leads to death, accompanied by
increased energy expenditure, decreasing weight and a loss of control of body temperature. However, most insomniacs never experience this total, devastating loss of sleep.

To sum up

There is no strong evidence that chronically disturbed sleep by itself causes ill health,
though you should be careful if you are driving or operating dangerous equipment:
however, there is no doubt that quality of life is reduced. Disturbed sleep reduces the
pain threshold, making pain less tolerable. People become irritable and concentration is
reduced. The loss of control may aggravate or promote various mental illnesses. But
is sleep good for you? It may not be. Death occurs most frequently around 09:00,
particularly from heart attacks. The cause is not clear, but is thought to be associated
with the increased load on the heart caused by getting up. Blood clots form more readily when your posture changes from lying down to standing up. And Mark Twain did
remark that beds were not a safe place to be, as so many people died in them!

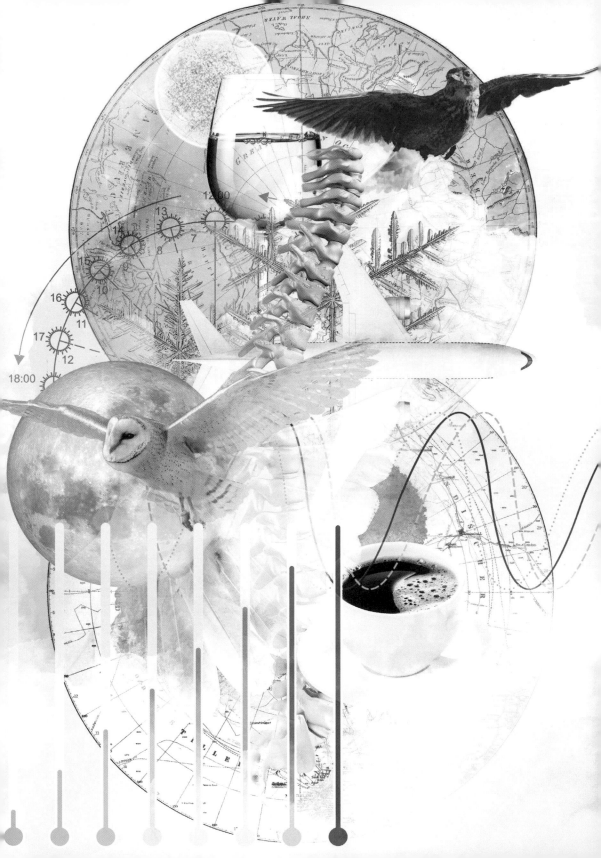

CHAPTER THREE

Managing your sleep

· ·

Chapter One introduced the idea that three processes controlled sleep: the sleep system, the awake system and the biological clock. Sleep is not just a process of letting go, but three processes working together; the sleep process taking over more and more of the brain with the awake process decreasing its grip and the biological clock having a permissive role. The biological clock provides a window of opportunity for either sleep or awake processes to dominate. It can cause certain disorders when it runs at the wrong speed, making people go to bed later and later (adolescents and young adults are more prone to this), or earlier and earlier (older people have more problems with this). The clock can also run at just slightly the wrong pace or the cues that synchronize it may not exert a strong enough effect. Cues include light, feeding, physical activity, work and social activity. One reason why elderly people may go to bed progressively earlier and earlier is that they do not go outside enough, or get enough natural light from windows, to help keep their biological clocks set at the right time.

Early-morning person (lark) or late-evening person (owl)?

Some people prefer to work late, go to bed late and wake up late. There is a strong genetic influence on which type you are. These people are referred to as 'owls'. Others are just the opposite, preferring to get up early, start work early and go to bed early. These people are called 'larks'. The questionnaire below helps you identify whether you are a morning person (lark) or an evening person (owl). Nowadays this is known as your 'chronotype'. You probably already know, but it is worth checking all the same, as the advice that relates to biological clock timing later on in the book needs to be considered in relation to which one you are.

Lark or owl?

Questions	Yes	No
Do you prefer to get up early in the morning (before 06:00)?		
Do you prefer to go to bed early (before 21:00)?		
Do you find it easy to go to bed at 21:00?		
Do you find it hard to stay up until 23:00?		
Do you usually become alert very quickly in the morning?		
Do you consider yourself a morning person?		

If you answered more than three of the questions yes then you could consider yourself a morning person.
If you answered more than three of the questions no then you could consider yourself an evening person.

The ruler on the page opposite, above, illustrates the bedtimes and rise times that extreme larks and owls could have. There is no research to show whether owls and larks are likely to become partners or not! The important point is that if owls go to bed too soon relative to their clocks, they will spend a long time going to sleep. Also, if they have to get up between 06:00 and 08:00 in the morning, they will end up feeling they have not slept well enough or for long enough. They could well end up thinking that they are insomniacs.

Larks could try to force themselves to stay up later in the evenings, but are still likely to wake up early. Again, they too could misunderstand the situation and believe that they have a sleep problem.

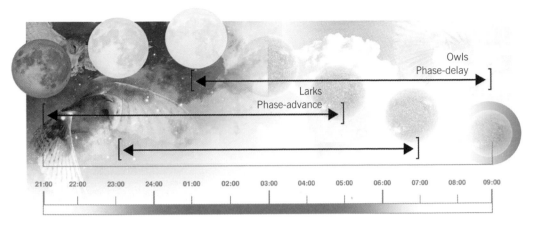

There are distinct sleep patterns between larks (advanced sleep) and owls (delayed sleep). So if you have trouble sleeping, it may just be that you are not sleeping at the right time relative to your clock.

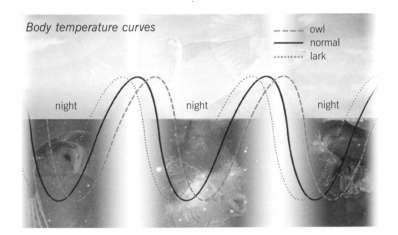

It is possible that body temperature curves run at different times in morning and evening types, as shown here.

Most people can appreciate the problems experienced by extreme larks and owls, because movement across two or three time zones affects most people. When the clocks are changed in spring and autumn (daylight saving), many people have adjustment problems for several days afterwards.

The illustration above shows the possible body temperature curves that morning and evening types may have. It is still not clear precisely how the clock system is affected: whether it runs particularly slowly in evening types and quickly in morning types, or whether it just runs at slightly different times in relation to light and dark.

Sleeping habits around the world

A study of sleep patterns around the world shows how sleep habits can adapt to different circumstances. In developed countries, the transition from an agricultural to an industrial economy and introduction of street lighting has caused many changes. Shiftwork, the move towards an early-morning work start time, the development of the nuclear family unit, the separation of children from the parental or grandparental sleeping environment and obesity have all contributed to considerable changes in sleep.

Yale University's Cross-cultural Survey (1937) noted the habits in siesta cultures throughout the world. In Patagonia: 'The Yahgans sleep together as a group and frequently interrupt each other's sleep … a tired person will lie down for a nap anywhere and at any time.' Comparisons of napping across siesta cultures show striking similarities: napping takes place mainly in the afternoon between 14:00 and 16:00; the length of the naps ranges between 1½ and 2 hours; nearly 90 per cent of napping cultures are found at latitudes between 30° North and 30° South – the more tropical the climate, the greater likelihood that napping occurs. This is another example where temperature is involved in the control of sleep.

Daylight extremes

Towards the North and South Poles, daylight times become more extreme, increasing in summer until there is continuous light and decreasing in winter until there is no sunlight at all. Not surprisingly, because of the effects of light on the biological clock, this has a major effect on sleep and on sleep-related disorders such as depression. A recent study in Svalbard, Norway – the most northern settlement in the world – examined how two ethnically different populations, native Norwegians and immigrant Russians, coped with the Arctic extremes of almost three months continuous daylight and over 2 months of complete darkness. Approximately 79 per cent of the Russians had sleep problems, compared with 24 per cent of the Norwegians. The Russians had more sleep problems during the polar night. Depression, dealing with shiftwork and inability to concentrate were common problems among both groups. Loneliness and alcohol consumption affected the Norwegians more than the Russians, who also noted worries as one of the causes of not sleeping well.

A circumpolar Siberian tribe, the Chukchi, were also observed from 1919–21 in a study by Yale University: 'As the nights were growing lighter the irregular habits of the Chukchi became almost intolerable [because of] their complete disregard for all division of time … One day they would sleep till noon, and would not crawl into their skins until midnight, get up, eat and go to sleep again in the morning. Day or night were ideas which no longer existed …'

Sleeping environment

Take a look at your sleeping environment as there are various aspects of it that will have an effect on your sleep. The main factors are listed below.

Light

Babies become infants, infants become children and so on. During this time a strong association between darkness and sleep is learned. For some people this association is not important for sleep, but for others, whose sleep has become fragile, light is one of the factors that needs to be controlled. It is worth seriously considering thick curtains or effective blinds, or both. Aluminium foil is a cheap, portable and temporary alternative. For those who have problems waking up in the morning, there are clocks with especially bright lights that strengthen the light of dawn. Light also exerts a strong influence via the biological clock (*see page 58*).

Noise

Hearing is actively turned down with the onset of sleep. Transmission of information from the ears to the auditory processing centres is reduced, but processing does not stop altogether. The brain's reaction to noise can be seen, when sleep is recorded using an EEG machine. Early research showed that the more salient and important the auditory information, the greater the brain's reaction – to the point that the person might wake up and be consciously aware of the noise. The noise of passing vehicles during sleep causes both a change in heart rate and a reaction in peripheral bloodvessels without necessarily awakening the sleeper or their being conscious of the noise. Nevertheless, the sleep is disturbed. The noise continues to act as a stress. A common observation among holiday-makers who go from a city environment to a quiet rural location is how much better they sleep, even if they are in different beds. Double- or triple-glazing is a general solution. Earplugs are a possible alternative. There is an obvious danger with earplugs, however, which is that alarms may not be heard.

Noise is a problem in many hospitals, particularly in intensive care units, and the healing process would be helped if natural sleep were promoted. So far, efforts have generally failed because of the practical difficulties, but eye masks and earplugs do help. Research has shown that in neonatal intensive care units, babies with a very low birth weight sleep more deeply and cry less if 'quiet hours' are introduced. The implication is that their sleep-awake cycles and general physiological stability are increased if these measures are adopted. Aircraft noise can definitely affect EEG, indicating lighter sleep. There is inconsistent evidence of other effects: higher psychiatric hospital admission rates, visits to doctors, self-reported health problems and use of medications. House insulation would help reduce noise, but not necessarily vibration. Mattresses will absorb vertical vibrations, but, depending on type, they may amplify as well as reduce horizontal vibrations. Even quiet traffic noise of 50dB, when accompanied by vibrations, is more disturbing than when there is just noise. REM sleep is more affected than other stages. Performance the following day can be impaired.

There have been attempts to make sleep more productive by learning something such as a foreign language, playing audio-tapes through specially adapted pillows. Unfortunately, the evidence suggests that it is only possible to learn material during the night if it wakes you up!

Safety

Many people complain that safety is a concern that prevents them from sleeping. This is difficult to deal with, as sleep has probably evolved to allow for occasional checking of the environment, and this may be one of the reasons for the ultradian cycle (*see pages 32–3*). Safety can refer to both physical and mental states. If the surroundings can be improved so as to provide a safer environment that in turn relaxes the individual, then sleep should improve. If safety of the psyche is the problem, then using the services of a cognitive psychotherapist would deal with this more directly. In the meantime, the thought-blocking exercises and mental relaxation exercises (*see pages 125–27*) in this book could also be used. If safety has been an issue for some time, there is a possibility that conditioned insomnia has also developed (*see pages 134–35*). Conditioning is enhanced with stress: post-traumatic stress disorder is the extreme case of this.

Bedroom temperature

It is impossible to dictate the correct temperature as this is a combination of the sleeper's own temperature, what the sleeper is wearing, bedclothes and also the ambient temperature. Cooler temperatures are generally appropriate, but extremes should be avoided. Overheating may not only disturb sleep, possibly with adverse daytime consequences, but may also damage the skin. As most couples will know, bed and bedroom temperature are sensitive issues. As little as half a degree difference can lead to a lively and non-sleep promoting environment.

Benjamin Franklin thought it was impossible to sleep when too hot, so he used two beds in a cold bedroom. When he found himself too hot in one bed, he would move to the other. Churchill, whose sleeping behaviour was quite unusual anyway, also preferred to have two beds, but in his case he preferred sleeping in an unwrinkled bed so he could move to a fresh bed when he had rumpled the first one!

Beds

Getting the right bed and pillow is important for a good night's sleep. If you wake up with aches and pains that disappear without treatment in one or two hours then it might be the sleeping surface that is causing the problem. Ideally, mattresses should make uninterrupted contact and distribute pressure evenly across the body. Hard mattresses have limited contact points, usually bottom and shoulders, so that pressure may lead to numbing and pain. Soft mattresses provide continual body contact but the neck and spine can sag, causing muscle tension and pain in some individuals (if you can sleep in a hammock or on a water mattress then a soft mattress will not trouble you).

Pillows should support your neck as well as your head. This is achieved by filling the space between neck and mattress, maintaining a straight line between the neck and spine. A specially designed posture support pillow may achieve this. It is helpful if hypoallergenic material is used for pillows and mattresses, as runny and stuffy noses or asthma can disturb sleep sufficiently to cause daytime performance problems. In schoolchildren this could manifest itself either as poor school performance or poor behaviour. According to a German proverb: *The best pillow is a clear conscience.*

Sleeping posture

It is possible to fall asleep in many positions, but some may lead to aches and pains. Your spine is aligned when you sleep on your side or back, but it is twisted if you sleep on your stomach, perhaps with one leg drawn up, bent at the knee. Misalignment may eventually occur, leading to muscle tension and pain. There are various patented pillows with built-in head and neck support that claim to keep your spine aligned. If in doubt, consult a chiropractor or osteopath.

Bed alignment was seen as significant by the author Charles Dickens. He carried a compass on his journeys so that he could align his bed north to south – he thought that the flow of magnetic current would benefit the sleeper.

Sleeping together

It is not unusual to find people sleeping in all kinds of places and in all sorts of positions, either alone, as couples or in groups. As long as the situation is not dangerous, and as long as you wake up feeling OK, are not stiff and do not fall asleep involuntarily during the day, then there is nothing to worry about.

In the West, the double bed is almost universal and it is regarded as normal for couples to sleep together. However, this has not necessarily always been the case, as this quotation from Dr James Graham in 1775 shows:

There is not in my opinion anything in nature which is more immediately calculated totally to subject health, strength, love, esteem, and indeed everything that is desirable in the married state, than that odious, most indelicate, and most hurtful custom of man and wife continually *pigging* together, in one and the same bed. Nothing more unwise – nothing more indecent – nothing more unnatural, than for a man and a woman to sleep, and snore, and steam, and do everything else that's indelicate together, three hundred and sixty-five times – every year.

Sleeping together is simply variable and depends a great deal on the culture. American children sleeping in the same bed would be regarded as unusual and most would find it desirable to sleep in their own bed, in their own bedroom. In contrast, Polynesian children would consider themselves abused if they were forced to sleep in this way because sleeping together as a group is still the normal practice in their society.

Bedtime routines

Regularity in routine is the rule for good sleep. Every night the biological clock is resynchronized to the sleep-awake routine. Even minor changes in routine can have a negative effect on this synchronization. It is a common experience to lie in at weekends and then find it difficult to go back to school or work on the Monday. Assuming nothing else was done over the weekend to disturb sleep, the probable cause is desynchronization between the biological clock and the sleep-awake cycle.

Bearing in mind that light exposure in the evening tends to slow down the biological clock and light exposure in the morning tends to speed it up, an extended time in bed in the morning will reduce the normal speeding up of the clock and thus delay the rhythm. This, coupled with the reduced time spent awake before trying to sleep, will lead to reduced sleep pressure and trying to sleep at a time when the biological clock will still be set for remaining awake. Even if you fall asleep, the clock will allow you to sleep longer the following morning, so when the alarm goes off you will find that you are sleepier than usual.

Menarche, menstruation, pregnancy and menopause

Every survey conducted shows that women suffer from disturbed sleep more than men. There are many reasons why, but the changes in hormonal status when periodic menstruation first begins (menarche), during the menstrual cycle and finally when menstruation ends (menopause) may contribute to this difference. Other factors that arise from childcare, such as breast-feeding and the distribution of parental work-load, may provide a background of sleep disturbance that eventually manifests itself as a long-term problem.

Not all women of reproductive age suffer from severe sleep difficulties, but many experience some change. Women who do not suffer from premenstrual syndrome symptoms can still take longer to fall asleep, wake more often and feel less refreshed after sleep during the luteal phase of the cycle. Sleep laboratory studies show subtle changes in sleep even in women who do not have any subjective awareness of any change. These changes involve an increase in the number of sleep spindles (patterns on the EEG), which peak during the luteal phase. The changes occur in parallel to the changes in core body temperature.

The 'rhythm method' of fertility control uses body temperature as one of its guiding factors and temperature affects sleep. This method can be very effective, but the change in temperature at the time of ovulation is similar in magnitude to the daily variation in most women. This makes it essential to measure temperature at the same time daily. Women who cross time zones or who are shift-workers may not only find difficulties in identifying accurately the time of ovulation, but their sleep may also be disturbed.

In pregnancy there are obvious changes in body weight and shape. In addition, in the third trimester the increased load on the heart and vascular system can lead to an increase in urine output that invariably disturbs sleep. There are huge hormonal changes during pregnancy, all of which have varying effects on sleep. In the first trimester, the feeling of fatigue may be caused in part by these hormonal changes.

Diet and drugs

Being overweight often causes problems with breathing, which may disturb sleep. The disturbance may not be great, but may be sufficient to disrupt sleep and cause daytime sleepiness.

The hormones insulin and cholecystokinin are released in the bloodstream after eat-ing. The insulin causes a fall in blood-sugar levels, which probably brings about feelings of tiredness. Cholecystokinin has a direct effect on the brain, promoting a feeling of satiation and sleepiness. For night-time sleep there is evidence that eating small amounts of light food shortly before going to bed may make some people feel comfort-ably full and help them go to sleep. Obviously, it is particularly important that the food is easily digested – anything that is heavy or likely to cause indigestion is not going to help. Fewer calories are burned up while you are asleep, so weight-watchers should not eat before going to bed, whereas those who want to put on weight could.

Caffeine

Caffeine increases alertness and undoubtedly disturbs sleep. Differences in metabolism, even differences with age, all create considerable variability in how caffeine will affect an individual. What is surprising is how many people are addicted to caffeine. Try stopping for a day – if you end up with a headache and feel sleepy, you are addicted!

This naturally occurring substance can be found in the leaves and seeds of more than sixty plants worldwide, the most common sources being coffee and cocoa beans, cola nuts and tea leaves. It is added to many foodstuffs and drinks, so it is not just consumption of tea and coffee that should be watched.

Caffeine is readily absorbed and peak concentrations occur in young adults 30–60 minutes after eating or drinking it (but illness or age widens the range to 15–120

FACTORS AFFECTING CAFFEINE METABOLISM

- *Exercise:* Moderate exercise increases the blood levels of caffeine, but also speeds up its metabolism.
- *Heredity:* Caffeine metabolism is controlled by many genes and racial differences exist.
- *Pregnancy:* In late pregnancy caffeine remains in the bloodstream for two and a half to seven times as long. There are no placental barriers to caffeine, so the foetus is exposed to its effects. In pre-term infants caffeine is only cleared out of the blood very slowly.
- *Disease:* Liver disease decreases caffeine metabolism.

Substances that reduce metabolism and clearance:
- Grapefruit juice *(not other citrus fruits; this is specific to grapefruit)*
- Oral contraceptives
- Cimetidine
- Disulfiram
- Alcohol
- Idrocilamide

Substances that increase metabolism and clearance:
- Smoking/enzyme inducers
- Rifamprin

minutes). It stays in the bloodstream for several hours, its concentration being reduced by half 3–5 hours after intake. Caffeine levels in the brain parallel that in the bloodstream, but if high doses are taken it may remain in the brain for 9–15 hours. Children tend to metabolize caffeine more quickly, as do smokers. This tolerance to caffeine not only varies over life but also varies with use. It is easy to get the shakes after too much caffeine if you have not had any for a while.

It is a powerful stimulant, but extensive research has not linked moderate consumption with any health problems, such as cancer, heart disease or infertility, nor does it appear to affect the development of the growing foetus. Nevertheless, it does show powerful effects on the brain.

The amount of caffeine in coffee depends on both the bean and the way it is prepared. Tanzanian Peaberry, Colombian and Indian Mysore beans have the highest percentage of caffeine; Mocha Mattari (from Yemen) and Mexican Pluma Altura have the lowest.

Guaraná

Guaraná (*Paullinea cupana*) is a tropical plant, grown in the Amazon region, which produces a small red fruit with a high caffeine content. It is chewed or dried and the powder dissolved in water. The European Medicines Agency Committee on Herbal Medicinal Products (HMPC) concluded that its seeds can be used in adults for the relief of symptoms of fatigue (tiredness) and weakness. The urban Brazilian version is a popular soft drink – insomniacs beware!

Alcohol

In small doses alcohol can reduce anxiety and promote sleep. It does not cause sleep – although larger doses may lead to unconsciousness and death – but it may aid the onset. It is estimated that 11 million Americans (6 per cent of the adult population) use alcohol to promote sleep. The rate of alcoholism in insomniacs is twice that of good sleepers and 60 per cent of alcoholics use alcohol as a sleep aid. There is evidence that a sleep disorder usually exists prior to the development of alcoholism. Consequently it has been estimated that 9–10 per cent of alcoholism is a consequence of insomnia.

Alcohol impairs breathing so it often causes further breathing problems for patients suffering from sleep apnoea (*see page 139*). Middle-aged males who snore and are sleepy during the day should be particularly wary of drinking alcohol as a sleep aid. A headache the following morning may be associated with impaired breathing during the night than the alcohol and its metabolites. Alcohol is also a diuretic, so part of the problem of waking up in the middle of the night after drinking alcohol is its effect on the kidneys. Finally, some people are particularly sensitive to alcohol, so only 1–2 glasses a night can disturb their sleep later in the night! (Note that alcohol is not legal in all jurisdictions.)

Nicotine

Nicotine is addictive and causes respiratory difficulties. Both can lead to sleep disturbance. Withdrawal is associated with headaches and sleepiness as well as increased appetite and weight gain.

Marijuana

Tetrahydrocannabinol (THC) is the active compound in marijuana. It may aid anxiety reduction and thus cause sleepiness indirectly. It takes longer to go to sleep after long-term use. It is illegal in many jurisdictions (as are the drugs in the following three entries).

Cocaine and crack

Cocaine is a stimulant that produces euphoria. It works through the brain messenger (neurotransmitter) dopamine, which is involved in the control of movement and wakefulness. Cocaine withdrawal is associated with sleepiness, which may persuade the individual to take more in order to function properly.

Amphetamines ('speed')

Amphetamines are powerful stimulants that work by changing the levels of several neurotransmitters including dopamine. Dopamine is altered in schizophrenia and this link is probably involved in the development of amphetamine psychosis. Amphetamine withdrawal is associated with increased sleepiness as well as increased REM during sleep. The increase in REM may be associated with nightmares.

Heroin

Heroin affects the pattern of sleep stages, but is most disturbing when it is discontinued. Intense nightmares may occur with the increase in REM found in withdrawal.

Sleep aids

Sleep aids that can be bought at pharmacies include pharmaceuticals, herbals, natural products and food supplements. Herbals, natural products (including melatonin) and food supplements are reviewed in Chapter Eight.

Over-the-counter aids

Pharmaceutical preparations generally contain sedating antihistamines, of which diphenhydramine is the most common. Diphenhydramine was developed to alleviate allergies and the fact that it caused sleepiness was initially regarded as a side effect. Subsequently, its use as an aid to sleep has become much more widespread although, unlike prescribed sleeping pills, high doses will not necessarily cause sleep. However, it has been used successfully as a sleep aid over many years without major incident or any major problems of dependence.

When writing this book the first time, it was not known how diphenhydramine worked. Histamine was not regarded as a neurotransmitter. With the discovery of the neuropeptide orexin, which is located in the 'awakening' centre of the brain, it was also found that it affected brain histamines. So it seems that diphenhydramine which penetrates the blood-brain barrier acts as an anti-wakefulness medicine. It promotes sleep by blocking the output of the wakefulness centre. So, if the sleep centre isn't active, sleep will not take place.

These sleep aids have two main problems: they take a long time to be cleared from the body and it is not obvious whether their effects dwindle over time. The directions on the label will usually tell the user to take these pills only at night-time and generally this should be OK (though some people may metabolize the pills slowly, so should be careful that they are not impaired in the morning). However, in my experience many people also wake up in the middle of the night and take these pills. This is very ill-advised as they are then likely to impair their performance and cognitive abilities the following day.

Prescribed sleeping pills

Generally, the advice on taking sleeping pills to cope with life stresses is – don't. It is a definite *do not* if the stress is likely to be chronic and recurring. There is also doubt whether sleeping pills are useful for a stress such as bereavement as there is evidence that it only delays the necessary bereavement process.

There are several types of sleeping pill available: barbiturates, benzodiazepines and 'non-benzodiazepines benzodiazepines' (the 'z' drugs) (*see box on the next page*). Barbiturates are very effective sleeping pills, as effective as a shotgun to the head – they are used as anaesthetics by veterinarians to put animals to sleep. However, they are dangerous in overdose, particularly when used with other drugs, and provide one of life's sometimes revolving exit doors (Marilyn Monroe and Jimi Hendrix are two famous examples of celebrities who died as a result of misusing these drugs).

Benzodiazepines are regarded as safe in contrast to barbiturates as they do not stop respiration in overdose. However, they are not 'pure' sleeping pills as they are also muscle relaxants, cause short-term amnesias and, more usefully, are anti-convulsants (anti-epileptic). Problems can emerge with benzodiazepines primarily if they are used long-term. They invariably cause rebound (increased) wakefulness after short-term use, which can lead to problems of withdrawal and addition. The 'non-benzodiazepine benzodiazepines', such as zolpidem, are newer compounds that affect the same sites in the brain as the benzodiazepines, but are not in the same chemical class.

Research continues on identifying a 'sovereign panacea' with close examination of the brain's own controlling mechanisms. For example, suvorexant, an orexin antagonist and so a wakefulness blocker, is an example of a completely new type of sleeping pill. In the meantime, and in parallel, the field of sleep disorders medicine continues to advance, with more and more causes being identified. Treatments can become more specific as causes are discovered.

DRUGS USED AS SLEEPING PILLS

Non-benzodiazepine benzodiazepines:
Imidazopyridines and Cyclopyrrolones
Short-acting, low daytime sedation.

Benzodiazepines
All benzodiazepines have been associated with dependence after long-term high-dose use. National regulatory authorities almost invariably advise short-term use only.

Chloral Derivatives
May cause high dose-dependence. Risk of gastric irritation and overdose.

Barbiturates
Risk of overdose, high dose-dependence, daytime sedation, biochemical tolerance.

Chlormethiazole
Risk of high dose-dependence. Associated with nasal irritation and confusion.

Antihistamines
Some toxicity in overdose, residual sedation. Can disturb normal sleep.

Antidepressants
Some have a soporific effect. Older tricyclics are toxic in overdose. Invariably disturb normal sleep, especially serotonin re-uptake inhibitors.

Antipsychotics
Risk of movement disorders makes antipsychotics, such as chlorpromazine, inappropriate for hypnotic use.

New drugs
The first orexin antagonist suvorexant (Belsomra) was registered in the US in 2014 and is currently available there and in Japan. Its mechanism of action is quite different to previous sleeping pills as it blocks the brain's promoting pathways at source.

DRUGS THAT AFFECT SLEEP

Non-psychotropic drugs
- Appetite suppressants
- Antiemetic drugs
- Antihistamines
- Corticosteroids
- Cardiovascular drugs
- Hormones and
  vitamin A

Psychotropic drugs
- Tricyclic and tetracyclic
  antidepressants
- Monoamine uptake
  inhibitors
- Monoamine oxidase
  inhibitors and reversible
  monoamine oxidase
  inhibitors
- Antipsychotics
- Anticonvulsants
- Hypnotics and
  stimulants

Recreational drugs
- Nicotine
- Alcohol
- Caffeine
- Herbs

Drugs of abuse
- Cannabinoids
- Hallucinogens
- Anabolic steroids
- Cocaine
- Heroin
- MDMA
- Amphetamine

Lifestyle

Unfortunately for all couch potatoes, moderate exercise has a beneficial effect on sleep. A recent study in the elderly (over 65s) found that exercise consisting of four 30–40 minute sessions of brisk walking a week was enough to improve sleep quality, the time it takes to go to sleep and sleep duration. Another study in a slightly depressed group aged between 60 and 84 examined the effects of a moderate weight-lifting program. These seniors engaged in their new exercises three times a week. Not only did their sleep improve over the 10-week period they were assessed, but also their depression lessened and other quality-of-life measures improved. Early evening exercise may be helpful because it helps maintain general fitness and the drop in body temperature after exercise may promote sleep.

Pre-sleep rituals

As sleep is partly a conditioned process, any routine that is associated with going to bed to sleep is to be encouraged – putting the cat out, locking up, cleaning your teeth and so on.

Hot baths

Hot baths are often suggested and are worth thinking about. Baths have been advocated for their mental and physical relaxation properties for many years, but the sleep researcher's perspective is different. It is thought that a bath causes a reactive decrease in body temperature, which promotes sleep. People with cold hands may also benefit. Their blood vessels are often constricted, so when the brain tries to open them up to release heat they refuse to work. A hot bath can help loosen them up, but so can a hand bath!

A nightcap?

As mentioned before, alcoholic nightcaps are to be avoided, or the amount should be small. Surprisingly little research has been done on the effects of non-alcoholic bedtime drinks. In the 1930s, two US researchers compared the effects on sleep of easily digestible snacks, such as cornflakes and milk, with less digestible snacks. They found that sleep was less restless with the easily digestible snacks. At the same time Nathaniel Kleitman, one of the founders of modern sleep research, found that Ovaltine, whether made with water or milk, was associated with more restful sleep compared to other snacks. Since then, Horlicks has been examined at the sleep laboratory at Edinburgh University by Kirstine Adam. Initially, she found that Horlicks improved the sleep of middle-aged subjects but not young subjects. Subsequently, it emerged that subjects who habitually had a bedtime snack slept well after Horlicks or a nutritionally-equivalent meal, whereas subjects who did not usually have a snack slept best without anything. Habit is obviously important.

A cup of tea?

Many elderly people have a cup of tea before going to bed or when they wake up in the middle of the night. The tea can have an alerting effect, but if the ritual is part of the conditioned process of going to sleep it is possible that the alerting effect becomes irrelevant as it peaks after sleep has begun.

Why can't I fall asleep?

In the first edition of the International Classification of Sleep Disorders (1990) there is a diagnosis of 'Inadequate Sleep Hygiene' which I think is still useful in spite of later editions dropping the term. Its list of diagnostics features is a useful guide to behaviours that may inhibit good sleep. It is a list of things not to do and in brackets a short note on why:

- Do not nap more than two times each week (lessens the need for nocturnal sleep).
- Do not get up or go to bed at irregular times (prevents the biological clock system from synchronizing with the awake system).
- Do not spend extended amounts of time in bed (if awake, this causes inappropriate awake conditioning: if asleep, it reduces the need for sleep the following night and in some circumstances it can reduce the cyclicity of the clock).
- Do not routinely use alcohol, tobacco or caffeine just before bedtime (all of these can disrupt sleep).
- Do not take exercise too close to bedtime (this prepares the body for wakefulness, not sleep).
- Try to avoid exciting or emotionally upsetting activities too close to bedtime (they fire up the awake system, may induce muscle tension and prepare the body for action).
- Do not use bed for non-sleep (sex allowed) activities, such as TV, reading, studying or snacking (otherwise the bed and bedroom become associated, by a conditioning process, with wakefulness, not sleep).
- Do not sleep on an uncomfortable bed with a poor mattress, inadequate blankets and so on (environmental conditions must be conducive to sleep, particularly if other problems with sleep are developing).
- Do not allow the bedroom to be too bright, stuffy, cluttered, hot, cold or in some way non-conducive to sleep (the environment must be right for you; it should also be dark).
- Do not perform activities demanding high levels of concentration shortly before going to bed (they fire up the awake system).
- Do not use bed for mental activities such as thinking, planning or reminiscing (bed is for sleep, so do not condition yourself to remain awake).

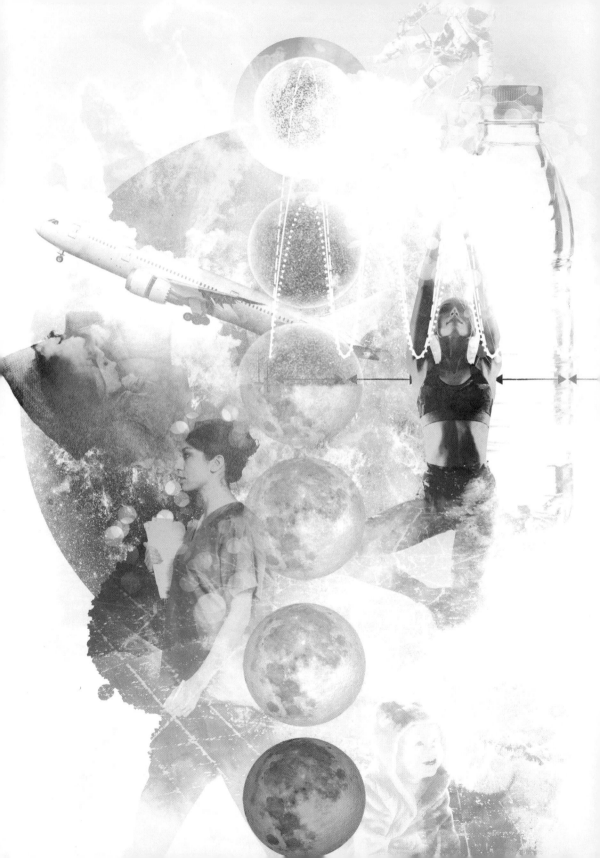

CHAPTER FOUR

Lifestyle and sleep

· ·

Life's various demands – children, the ill, the incapacitated, work, the commute, even holidays – all eat into our waking time, with the result that sleep is often neglected. For many of us, this does not cause a problem. Our genetic constitution, our general health, the adaptability of our sleep-awake systems and how they interact with our internal biological clock allow most of us to get sleep when we need it. But others are not so lucky.

For them, the biological clock is an important determinant of when they go to sleep and when they wake up, how alert they feel and how well they can do tasks. The biological clock's effect on alertness is much greater than is usually appreciated. It is not total, but a reasonable guestimate is that at least 50 per cent of people rely heavily on the clock running correctly. Even a 1-hour change in time, say for daylight savings, has a measurable effect on the population as a whole.

This chapter will look at jet lag and shiftwork first, because of the importance of appreciating the interactions between the sleep, awake and clock systems. Learning how to cope with these situations is a good primer for working out how to cope with situations when you cannot control your own sleep, or when you are acting as a carer.

Light and the biological clock

Charles Czeisler of the Harvard Medical School has conducted research for more than 40 years into the effects of light on circadian rhythms. He found that intense artificial light can shift the circadian (24-hour) rhythms that are controlled by the biological clock. The intensity of that light (10,000 lux for the technically minded) was much brighter than normal indoor light and is roughly equivalent to the amount of light needed to take a photograph with a cheap camera that does not have a flash. The effect is so powerful that Czeisler and Harvard have patented the use of light for medical purposes.

This remains one of the most important discoveries in sleep research. Before, it was not thought possible to rapidly change the timing of the clock. The diagram on page 61 illustrates the effect. If you are exposed to light prior to your body temperature minimum (say in the evening), this tends to force the minimum away from its usual time. In other words, you will wake up later. Conversely, if light (usually dawn) is present shortly after body temperature minimum, then the following night the minimum occurs earlier – you will fall asleep earlier. When I checked the original research paper it had been cited 553 times but more importantly, the application of the result has moved into the mainstream.

Enlightened architects (pun intended) will, for example, consider the effects of light, particularly blue light (*see no '2' in the list of new findings on page 9*) on people in a building. The original iPhones, iPads and tablets by chance emitted the blue light frequencies that most affected the biological clock. Apple and tablet manufacturers have since changed the frequencies so that their devices do not emit the light that affects the biological clock most.

Jet lag

Jet lag is a good example of how things go wrong with the biological clock. It is caused by moving to a new time zone faster than the clock can adapt. This can cause various problems, in particular difficulties with getting to sleep and staying asleep. This can be coupled with sleepiness during the day and stomach upsets. The severity of the problem varies with the number of time zones crossed and the direction. A flight of up to 3 hours westwards does not generally cause a big problem. Eastwards, though, and the problems begin to mount up. Getting to sleep, waking up, feeling well, feeling alert – nothing is as easy as it was. Make it a transatlantic or transpacific crossing (more than three time zones) and the problems really start to mount.

Jet lag can be sufficiently debilitating to cause problems with work or enjoying a holiday. Long plane trips can lead to dry, itching eyes, dry or runny noses, headaches, muscle cramps and various other symptoms of general malaise, but these are not representative of true jet lag. They are the direct effect of the flight.

Generally, individuals suffering from sleep problems get little sympathy. Sleep is regarded as one of those facets of behaviour that an individual can control at will. Jet lag, however, is a common problem experienced by many – and an ideal way for good sleepers to begin to appreciate how a chronically poor sleeper feels! The jet-lagged individual knows, at least, that the problem is not permanent.

Coping with jet lag

First, make sure that you take care of all the problems that may be caused by the flight itself:

- Use creams to keep your skin moist and your eyes and nose comfortable.
- If you are travelling low-budget economy, remember your eye-mask and earplugs.
- If you are tall, try to find out what plane you are likely to be flying on so that you can arrange a seat that gives you lots of leg room.
- Revise your favourite muscle-stretching exercises.
- If you find aeroplane seats uncomfortable, then buy a traveller's pillow or any other device that will help you maintain a comfortable posture.
- If you take medicines, consult with your doctor to check whether your flight might cause a problem. Also, find out how to handle the time-zone differences. Do you take an extra pill or one less?
- Do not take sleeping pills or buy over-the-counter sleep aids. Prescribed sleeping pills can be of short duration so theoretically could be used on a flight, but there are two main problems. First, if there was an emergency you might not be able to cope. Second, these pills cause amnesia: you can wake up under the influence, engage in activities and go back to sleep again. When you wake up again you may not be able to recall what you have done (or what you agreed to) when you were awake! Melatonin is the exception.
- Over-the-counter sleep aids that contain antihistamines (see page 51) stay in the brain far too long to be useful. You may sleep during the flight, but you might not cope with immigration or customs afterwards.
- Try to move your sleep towards the destination time before you leave, particularly if you have an important meeting. If travelling eastwards, go to bed and get up earlier each day for a few days before departure. Conversely, travelling westwards, you should try to move your sleep time later each day and get up later.

Diet

Try to adjust your diet so that eating is more closely timed to your destination time. A special diet had been advocated for many years by the US military. The Argonne diet involves alternating between fasting and feasting. The principle is to eat high-protein meals when you are trying to stay awake and high-carbohydrate meals when you want to be sleepy. The original study has never been properly repeated and it had methodological problems. But there is some newer supporting literature and experimental work looks promising. This diet is outlined below.

Before the flight

- Three days before the flight start eating high-protein breakfasts and lunches and high-carbohydrate suppers.
- Avoid caffeine (*see pages 48–9*) and other mild stimulants except for mid-afternoon.
- Two days before the flight reduce calorie intake to around 800 calories by keeping meals light. Keep the same balance of high-protein breakfast and lunch and high-carbohydrate supper. Do not eat any food after supper.
- On the day before the flight eat as much as you want, but keep the food balance the same and don't eat anything after supper.

The day of the flight

- This is similar to day 2 and is a low-calorie-intake day (800 calories). Maintain the same diet as before. On the flight, drink lots of water to combat dehydration. Remember, alcohol promotes dehydration. Even moderate dehydration can cause fatigue and listlessness.
- Set your watch to the destination time and just note how the airlines feed you at peculiar times.

After the flight (breakfast at your destination)

- Using destination time, get up half an hour before breakfast and do some light stretching exercises. Drink one to two cups of strong coffee between 06:00 and 07:30. Today, feast on a high-protein breakfast and lunch and high-carbohydrate supper. Avoid caffeine after breakfast and no naps during the day. Keep as active as possible.

Finding light and avoiding light

The beginning of this chapter focused on the effects of light on the biological clock. You can use this to speed up your adjustment to a new time zone. The important factor is how much light reaches your eyes. You can sit in the shade outside provided your eyes are getting the benefit of light. Sitting inside looking out of a window is fine. Generally, 2 or 3 hours difference eastward or westward causes few problems. Problems start from 4 hours onwards.

The most general advice to give when travelling east is that you should improve your adjustment by being outside in the morning and midday light. Travelling westwards, the middle and late afternoon light can help.

Two more examples may help. First, decide whether you are an owl or a lark (see page 40). If you are neither, and regularly get up at around 07:00 at home, you can assume that your body temperature minimum occurs around 04:00. Remember always to adjust your watch to the new time as soon as possible.

If you are travelling four time zones eastwards, then avoid light between 03:30 and 08:30 and then look for bright light until 11:30. If you travel four time zones westwards, you should look for bright light between 21:30 and 00:30, and then avoid bright light until 04:30 or later. Clearly, westwards is a problem unless you are staying at a hotel that can provide special bright lights (see 'Sleep-tight rooms' page 62).

These times need to be adjusted depending on your habitual wake-up time (and therefore your biological clock minimum). If, for example, you usually get up at 05:00,

The effect of light on the biological clock

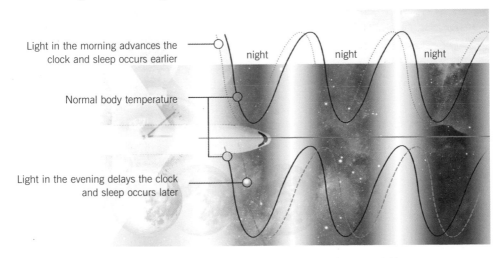

When you are travelling you can use light to help your biological clock adjust more quickly to your new time zone.

then the eastwards flight should be followed by avoidance of light between 01:30 and 06:30, and looking for bright light until 09.30. Similarly, a westward flight would be followed by looking for light between 19:30 and 22:30, and then avoiding light until 02:30.

'Sleep-tight' rooms

In the first edition of the book, the Hilton hotel group was described as having taken the problem of jet lag seriously. A number of its hotels boast 'sleep-tight' rooms, which were specially designed with the National Sleep Foundation to help adjust to time-zone changes. These rooms had special light boxes and lighting systems, white-noise machines or soothing CDs, special mattresses and pillows and earplugs. There was also a special two-call wake-up system for travellers who were not sleeping because they were worried that they might not wake up in time. Since then, other hotel groups have adopted similar measures. These come and go so it's necessary to check what your hotel does. Even budget hotels have recognized that special features make for happier customers.

Shiftwork

In 1991 the US Congress estimated that 60–90 per cent of Americans on shiftwork had sleep disorder problems. Little has changed since then. Shiftworkers are static time-zone travellers. They have to optimize their working efficiency, whatever shift they are on. There are no shiftsystems that cater for the problems of biological clock and sleep-awake adjustment. Apart from accidents partly caused by working at night on shift (such as Chernobyl, Three-Mile Island, Exxon Valdez – all extremely costly accidents), I originally wrote that shift systems did not appear to cause long-term health problems. However, I also said that this might be illusory, as people who couldn't tolerate shift systems would tend to leave their jobs. Vocational jobs such as nursing might end in failure because a person cannot adapt to working shifts. This self-selection would reduce the possibility of detecting whether health problems are developing.

Nurses have often been studied on shift systems. More than 40 years ago, it was noted that nurses whose body temperature curves were beginning to adapt to their shift system had less of a problem with shifts. The nurses whose biological clocks were difficult to change found shift systems more difficult. It was not known at that time that light could be a potent tool for changing the timing of the biological clock. This may also help others who have more difficulty in handling shift systems.

Larks, and people aged over 50, seem to have more problems handling shifts. Unfortunately, the situation is now worse. Our 24/7 societies have increased the number of people doing shiftwork, which is associated with metabolic disease. Metabolic disease is a mixture of type 2 diabetes, obesity and metabolic syndrome. This leads to cardiovascular disease, diabetes, musculoskeletal diseases, sleep apnoea and, in some circumstances, cancer. There are 1.9 billion adults, 39 per cent of the global adult population obese. It is estimated that 20 per cent of the Western workforce are engaged in shiftwork. Apart from trying to work at the wrong time relative to the biological clock, social and domestic commitments make life difficult for shiftworkers. The work environment often does not have extra bright lights for the nightshift worker and even going home after the nightshift means that light is re-synchronizing the clock to the wrong time. Once home, bedrooms are probably not adequately shielded and rooms may not be sufficiently sound-proofed. Double or triple glazing, double blinds and thicker doors can all improve sleep continuity and quality by increasing the efficiency of the sleep system. When shiftwork leads to intolerable insomnia or sleepiness it may be diagnosed as Shift-work Disorder (*see page 131*).

Dark goggles

Bright light can be effective in experimental conditions in delaying the biological clock and improving sleep. So, potentially, it can be useful for night-shift workers. One study has found that bright light in the workplace (up to around 04:00) can help delay the sleep-awake cycle, but the journey home from work in the dawn light (in other words, after the temperature minimum) is enough to reduce its effectiveness. The solution appears to be to use dark goggles, which are darker than normal sun-glasses. Blinds, possibly double blinds, to prevent light getting into the bedroom are also extremely important for the shiftworker trying to sleep.

It has been estimated that out of all the cues that might align the biological clock with the sleep-awake cycle (food, social cues, noisy children and so on), light might account for 70–90 per cent of the alignment signal.

What you should do

The answer varies depending on the shift-work scheme that you are on, what type of person you are on the lark/owl continuum, how old you are and what kind of sleeper you are. You need to identify these features in the various question and diary sections in this book.

NASA

Astronauts are put on a 24-hour day-night, awake-sleep cycle, but NASA has gone further in trying to improve the performance of its workforce. It has recognized that the best shiftwork schedules involve long-term adaptation and that this is impractical. Using natural cues can also be impractical. They have found that self-administered light of 10,000 lux at appropriate times of day phase-delayed circadian rhythms sufficiently to allow the workforce to parallel the activity demanded by the Space Shuttle missions. NASA subjects not only reported improved sleep and performance, but better physical and emotional wellbeing as well. A fatigue management team make sure they get their timing right!

Adolescents

Are adolescents and young people going to bed later and later? Survey results appear to indicate that this is the case. The ubiquitous presence of caffeine (*see pages 48–9*), smartphones and tablets, as well as many social factors will be helping young people to stay awake, but once they do, the biology of the sleep, awake and clock systems will conspire to make them sleepy and alert at the wrong times.

The brain's biological clock generally runs slowly and light towards the end of the day tends to slow it down even further. The melatonin secreted by the pineal gland will advance the clock, as will the dawn and morning light. However, if the youngster goes to bed late, the amount of time during which melatonin is secreted decreases (so the clock is advanced less) and they miss the early light (so again the clock is advanced less).

The upshot is that the clock remains delayed, so the youngster tends to go to sleep even later the following night. School or job demands will force them to get up the next morning, partially sleep-deprived and effectively jet-lagged.

The elderly

Napping increases as a person gets older. This may be due to a number of factors: changes in lifestyle; the development of sleep disorders that disturb sleep during the night and increase sleepiness during the day; because an intrinsic rhythm of the biological clock re-asserts itself or the biological clock itself is running differently or because various ailments of the elderly are disturbing their sleep.

Generally, napping should not be considered a problem, especially if the individual does not regard it as such. Note the sleep taken over a 24-hour period and count the nap as part of the total. If this equates to an amount similar to that when you were young, then there is probably no problem. If you were a 6-hour sleeper and you take a 1-hour nap during the day, then expect only 5 hours sleep during the night. There

Average sleep pattern in the elderly

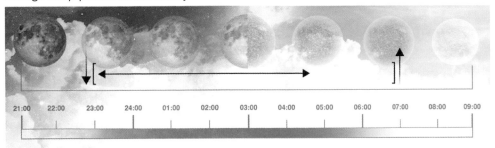

Earlier bedtime develops in the elderly

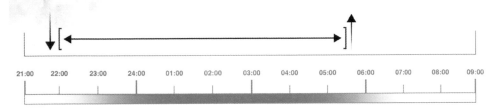

The rulers above show typical diaries for the elderly. The top one shows an early night but early morning awakening. The lower one shows an even earlier bedtime.

Daytime napping in the elderly

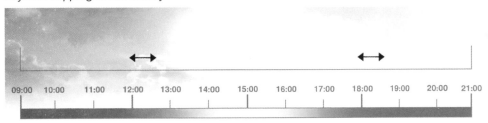

The earlier bedtime is also associated with daytime napping, as shown above.

may be a problem if the sleepiness during the day is uncontrollable (*see pages 136–37*) and particularly if the night's sleep is considered unrefreshing.

The diagram above illustrates one of the problems that the elderly may have if they no longer go out much. Many elderly people go to bed earlier and wake up earlier, which may reflect a slight change in their biological clock time. If they also do not go out as much, it means that the synchronizing effects of light on the biological clock are reduced. This means that amplitude – the measure from peak to trough – is also reduced. This reduction in amplitude coupled with a slight drift to higher overall average means that

Biological clock in the elderly

The elderly tend not to go out as much, meaning that the effects of light on the biological clock are reduced. Sleep is therefore not as deep, more easily disturbed and length of sleep is shorter.

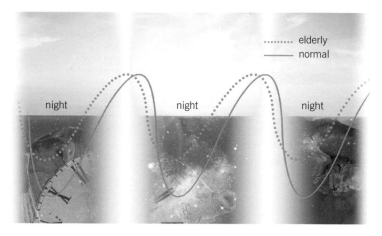

sleep will not be as deep, will finish earlier and will be more prone to upset. The solution is to try to use ambient light, if not the specialist bright lights used by NASA, to enhance the amplitude of the rhythm. Just going outside in the evening light, or sitting in front of a window may do – it will indirectly strengthen sleep.

When your work demands that you stay awake

Doctors and nurses are more likely to be involved in road accidents when driving home if they have been working for extended periods. If you abuse your sleep, your subsequent alertness will also be abused. Nevertheless, emergencies, illness, staffing levels and so on may lead to the need for medical, nursing and auxiliary staff to work long hours. How do they cope in these circumstances?

Being aware of the dangers of unintended sleepiness is a first step. Most people can overcome sleepiness for short periods of time. The dangers are associated with boring and monotonous tasks, such as highway driving. Naps do provide a great benefit. The longer the nap, the greater the benefit. Caffeine is also a remarkably good stimulant and will make people alert, even though they may not feel well.

Core versus optional sleep

When I was looking at the effects of sleep on memory, I ran an experiment that allowed the volunteers varying durations of sleep with little control of the sleep stages. The study was EEG controlled, so subjects were woken up when a cycle of sleep had completed (this would be at peak alertness on the ultradian cycle shown on page 69). Surprisingly, the stages of sleep were less important than the duration. The longer the subjects slept, the better their memory. Since then, Jim Horne (Loughborough, UK) has suggested that the first three or four cycles of sleep are essential to function properly (core sleep) and the rest is optional.

Rules for core sleep

Unfortunately, though this seemed a good idea, very little experimental data has emerged over the last 20 years to support it and restricted sleep, 4.5 hours approximately or less, over a period of weeks will have a deleterious effect on performance and wellbeing. Nonetheless, in emergencies the following strategies may be helpful (both shiftwork and jet lag might be regarded as 'emergency situations'):

* If you can, get at least 5 hours
* Anchor sleep
* Charge your sleep batteries
* Long naps
* Ultra-short sleeps.

Anchor sleep

Two UK researchers started investigating anchor sleep in the early 1980s. They divided an 8-hour sleep period into two 4-hour periods and kept one of those 4-hour sleep periods at the same time every day. They found that the circadian rhythms quickly re-established themselves if a period of anchor sleep was maintained and it didn't really matter when the other 4 hours of sleep occurred. The core-sleep quota could be managed by taking additional sleep at some other time during the day. For shiftworkers, this can be helpful, as they can choose an anchor-sleep period that is more or less constant across all their shifts. The minimum quota of core sleep can be achieved by having an anchor sleep and getting a second sleep some time over a 24-hour period.

Charging your sleep batteries

David Dinges in the US investigated prophylactic sleep – taking some extra sleep in advance of an anticipated period of sleep disruption. It is not clear whether this achieves a significant improvement in alertness during the period of sleep disruption, but it does appear to have some positive effects. Again, if the bottom diagram on page 69 is considered, a sleep (a nap) prior to normal sleep will reduce sleep pressure. If sleep pressure is reduced by a prophylactic nap, then alertness may benefit.

Long naps

In situations where sleep is being disturbed regularly and waking activity is taking priority, then any nap is probably better than none and the longer the nap, the better. If naps are difficult to get started, then some of the techniques in Chapter Six may be useful.

Ultra-short sleeps

In situations where sleep has gone wrong, the emphasis is on how fragmented the sleep has become and what impact this has on daytime functioning. However, if a person is a normal sleeper, someone who would sleep normally if circumstances allowed, then sleep fragmentation seems less significant. Just getting the sleep is important. It is not clear what the minimum should be: it might be as little as 4–10 minutes, but it certainly seems in the order of 30–40 minutes, not 3–4 hours. There is also some evidence that very short naps may prevent the rare but serious problem of 'freezing' – failing to respond in a serious situation instead of acting.

There are certainly problems to be aware of if you are having ultra-short sleeps, sleep inertia being the most important. Sleep inertia is a period of impaired performance that lasts between 5 and 20 minutes after waking up. It is a reality – US Air Force crews are prohibited from napping when on immediate alert or standby because of this fact. The recommendation is that anyone who needs an alert mind immediately on waking up should not take naps. Those who can afford to take a little longer to wake up could use the simple expedient of washing the face with cold water.

Napping and nappers

The top diagram (*opposite*) illustrates a normal night's sleep. Looking at the peaks, slow-wave sleep can be seen to decrease during the night. Slow-wave sleep is sometimes regarded as an index of sleep pressure. The decline is not continuous but oscillates. The slow-wave sleep troughs are punctuated by the 90-minute ultradian cycle.

The bottom diagram illustrates what happens after one night's sleep deprivation. The slow-wave sleep peaks are much higher and the decrease during the night is more rapid. Sometimes the ultradian cycle is also distorted and the slow-wave sleep cycles lengthen. Daytime napping has the opposite effect and decreases the peaks of the slow-wave sleep cycle. Slow-wave sleep is driven very precisely by the amount of preceding wakefulness before sleep onset. If slow-wave sleep is an accurate index of sleep pressure, it is obvious why sleep advisers always suggest that people should not nap

Slow-wave sleep and ultradian cycles

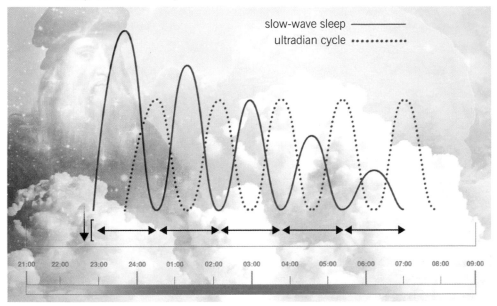

Slow-wave sleep after sleep deprivation or napping

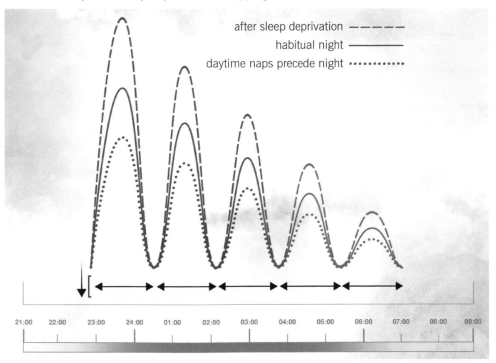

during the day. Reduced sleep pressure means that the interrupting ultradian cycle is more likely to leave someone wide awake when they wake up in the middle of the night than it would if overall sleep pressure was higher. On the other hand, if you are not worried about getting a continuous night's sleep and get a reasonable quota over a 24-hour period, there is no problem.

Claudio Stampi, a sleep researcher, has identified a number of famous nappers: Winston Churchill, Leonardo da Vinci, Napoleon, Salvador Dalí and Thomas Edison. He found that Leonardo da Vinci adopted a very unusual sleep-awake pattern. He would sleep for 15 minutes out of every 4 hours, giving a daily total of only 1½ hours! Stampi calculates that during da Vinci's 67 years he gained in effect almost an extra 20 years by adopting this unique pattern of sleep.

Carers

Babies, toddlers, the ill and the ailing elderly may demand so much of your time that you cannot manage a whole night's sleep. What do you do? Don't give up – there are various strategies you can adopt, including taking care of your core sleep, mentioned earlier in this chapter (*see page 67*).

Self-help for carers

Are you stressed by looking after someone else? The questions in the chart opposite provide an indication (tick the column that matches closest how you feel). If one or two ticks are in the 'Nearly always true' column then you might start to look for help with caring and help in taking care of yourself. In the meantime, the section called 'Pulling it all together' (*see page 72–3*) will try to help with your sleep.

More sleep facts

So far this book has talked about a sleep system, an awake system, a circadian (24-hour) clock system and an ultradian (90-minute) cycle. There are other ultradian cycles, and one of them runs every 12 hours. This became evident when volunteers were instructed to sleep for as long as possible. When they had slept around 12 hours the amount of slow-wave sleep started to increase (which didn't make a lot of sense as slow-wave sleep is promoted mainly by the duration of preceding wakefulness). This was evidence for a 12-hour cycle. Since then more evidence has emerged.

Peretz Lavie's 7/13-minute sleep-wake schedule has plotted what he called the sleep propensity function. The main feature is an increased ability to sleep during the

Caregiver's stress test

Questions	Seldom true	Sometimes true	Often true	Nearly always true
I find I can't get enough rest				
I don't have enough time for myself				
I feel guilty about my situation				
I don't get out much any more				
I have conflict with the person I care for				
I worry about having enough money to make to make ends meet				
I have conflict with other family members				
My own health is not good				
I cry every day				
I don't feel I have enough knowledge or experience to give care as well as I'd like				
I don't have time to be with other family members besides the person I care for				

night, but it also points to a 2-hour sleep cycle (possibly related to the 90-minute ultra-dian rhythm that has already been described) as well as an increased ability to sleep in the afternoon. He has also shown that there are specific, to use his term, 'gateways', into sleep. These gates can also close, creating 'forbidden zones'. The forbidden zones occur in the evening prior to sleep, whereas the gateways exist just before sleep.

These observations explain why a nap in the early evening may not disturb sleep. The nap presumably takes place at the peak of the 2-hour cycle. If sleep is then attempted at the usual time, which should coincide with the main nocturnal gate, then sleep will run its usual course through the night (although awakening in the morning might be a little earlier). If the main nocturnal gate is missed, then the individual may find that they have to wait until the next gateway opens up.

Knowledge of the gateways and the cyclical nature of sleep is helpful for those who have problems with their sleep. Their anxiety about sleep can to some extent be reduced if they know that remaining awake in these circumstances is natural.

Pulling it all together

Earlier in the book, I described how sleep was an active process that interacted with the demands of wakefulness and various time-driven rhythms. This knowledge can be used to optimize your sleep time.

You may not manage to catch up with your sleep every day, but hang on and try to catch up with your sleep at least once a week. As the main stages of sleep compensate for losses, one night in seven will allow you to catch up with a lot of the major sleep stages you have lost during the week. Staying in bed longer once a week can also help you recuperate without having an impact on your sleep in relation to the biological clock. You might be able to manage more than once a week, but if you start failing to sleep at your usual bedtime, then you should reconsider your strategy and limit the lie-in to once a week.

The recommendation not to nap (*see pages 68 and 70*) is aimed primarily at those whose sleep is already failing and out of control; it is not directed at those who have to survive on minimal amounts of sleep. Along with other researchers, I argue that sleep is probably set up to occur mainly during the night, but not exclusively, with some time being allotted to it during the day. You don't have to listen to me – just talk to anyone who still lives in a siesta culture.

An early study from the National Institute for Occupational Safety and Health found that naps significantly improve alertness, mood and job performance. It also showed that the best, most refreshing time to doze is mid-afternoon, some time between 13:00 and 16:00, coinciding with many of the observations already noted in this book. How long you should nap for, you will have to discover yourself. As noted earlier, some people dislike naps because they feel awful afterwards. We know that these people run a slightly higher body temperature, but we don't know the most effective way of counteracting the negative effects (although they are likely to feel better later in the day). Sleep inertia is a problem, so be wary after a nap, don't make vital decisions and don't drive if you can avoid it.

Evening naps may pose a problem for night sleep, but on the other hand, if you are desperate to catch your favourite television programme or remain conscious with your amorous partner, then an evening nap might be a lifesaver. Reading to children and then falling asleep for a short nap with them not only promotes a closer relationship but may also set you up for the night. Nap when the children nap. If they are cranky, but they do fall asleep in the car, take them out for a drive. When the children fall asleep, you might want to stop and try to get a nap yourself. (Always stop for a rest if you feel sleepy when driving, but remember, you may feel the effects of sleep inertia when you wake up.)

At work, a nap might be better than a coffee break if you can manage it. It partly depends what you need to do after the break. A nap may result in sleep inertia, but it will help you remain awake longer. Caffeine improves alertness very rapidly (within 20–30 minutes) and, depending on your metabolism, keeps you going for a couple of hours, but the downside is that you become dependent on it. If you think you need caffeine all the time, then you need to consider rescheduling your sleep another way. If you are a commuter, then take a nap on the train or bus, but use a travel pillow (or pocketbook, shopping bag, whatever) to support your head and if you have a travelling companion, get them to wake you up.

Alcohol is not a good idea. Use it as an occasional nightcap if you like, but be vigilant about how much you are drinking, and how often.

Exercise to maintain general fitness, but do not exercise close to bedtime. Once the body gets ready for action it tends to stay in that state for several hours. Do not be fooled if you fall asleep quickly after exercise; your sleep will be more disturbed and you will wake up less refreshed.

Finally, if your muscles are tense and you suffer from headaches, stomach aches, anxiety or depression, then you probably need to work on stress reduction. The fatigue may be stress-related rather than sleep-related.

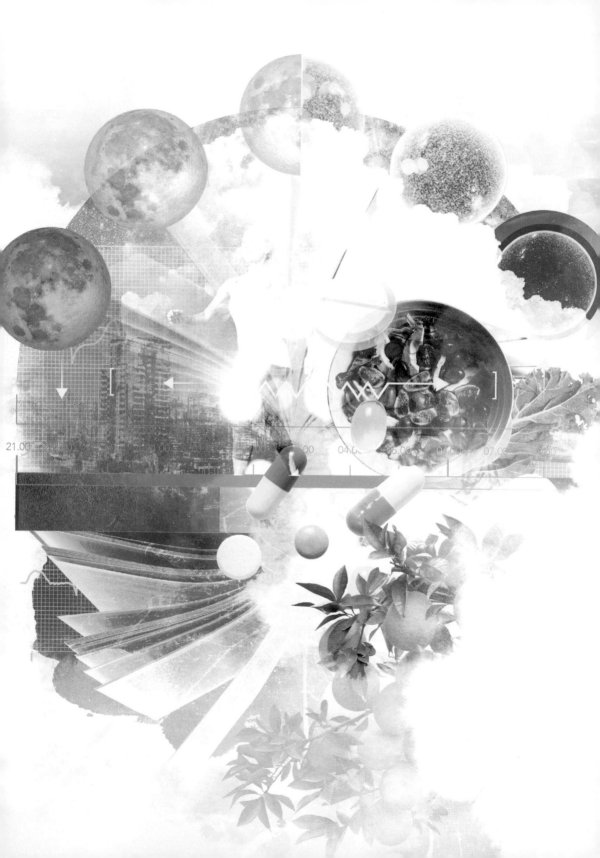

CHAPTER FIVE

The diary

. . . .

The diary and rulers are the most important part of the assessments because they enable you to monitor your sleep accurately, so that you can start to work out what is going on. The daily questions and rating scale focus on some attributes and are used later in the assessment.

How to fill in the diary

Let's have a brief recap on the rulers that were first introduced in Chapter Two and how to fill them in, then I'll take you through the different sections of the diary to show you how to complete your diary pages.

Filling in the diary and rulers should not disrupt your sleep and it is accepted that the readings may not be entirely accurate. You do not have to fill in the ruler during the night. And there is no need to stare at the bedroom clock. If you realize you are awake, mentally note the time and write it down in the morning. If you have to get up to attend to children, go to the lavatory, get a drink of water or whatever, then also note the time.

The night ruler

A completed night ruler is shown opposite, with a space for your abbreviations. This night ruler illustrates quite a nasty night. The person goes to bed (↓), then spends an hour reading. When he or she tries to sleep ([), it takes an hour to fall asleep (←), only to wake up 1½ hours later. About half an hour awake is followed by 3 hours of fragmented and troubled sleep (∿). The sleeper then drifts off for 1½ hours of tranquil and pleasant sleep (—), only to wake up (→) and spend another hour trying to sleep again. The night ends with an hour of doing something such as watching TV ( ]) before getting up (↑). If this is you, you are probably in trouble; on the other hand, you may just have been on a long-haul flight! Shown below is a list of abbreviations you could use to describe what you are doing during the night and day. The bad-night example is shown with abbreviations included. The night starts (or finishes) with some alcohol (A) and food (F). The first period awake in bed is spent reading (R). Sleep is broken by some interruption (I) – this could be noise, such as a baby crying, or being too hot or cold. Later on in the night there is a visit to the lavatory (L) and the night ends by watching morning television (T). More detailed notes and observations can also be written on the page and in the box provided (*see 'Notes and medication' overleaf*).

THE RATING SCALE: ACTIVITIES AND DISTURBERS		
A Alchohol	**E** Exercise	**P** Pain/Discomfort
C Caffeine	**D** Dreams	**W** Worries
F Food	**N** Nightmares	**T** Television/Radio
M Medicine	**I** Interruption	**In** Internet
S Smoking	**L** Lavatory	**R** Reading

NIGHT RULER I • Date:

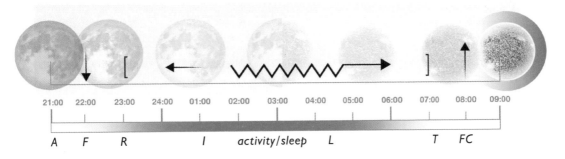

21:00	22:00	23:00	24:00	01:00	02:00	03:00	04:00	05:00	06:00	07:00	08:00	09:00

A   F   R   I   *activity/sleep*   L   T   FC

Complete promptly in the morning

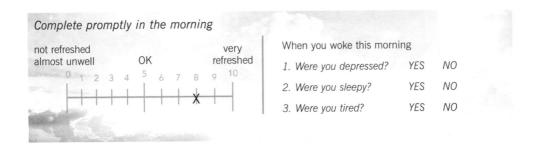

not refreshed
almost unwell   OK   very refreshed

0 1 2 3 4 5 6 7 8 9 10

When you woke this morning

1. Were you depressed?	YES	NO
2. Were you sleepy?	YES	NO
3. Were you tired?	YES	NO

The rating scale

Above, you will see the rating scale. It will help you to identify how you slept during the night and should be filled in within a few minutes of getting up. If you wake up feeling OK – neither tired and unrefreshed, nor really wide-awake or hyper – then put a cross on the scale below the 'OK'. If you are feeling really quite well and refreshed, then mark the scale a little higher, say 8 (*as shown*). On the other hand, if you are feeling only a little bit better than dead, mark the scale much lower, say 1 or 2! If you have had a bad night's sleep, then you won't be surprised to note that you feel unrefreshed. On the other hand, disorders such as sleep apnoea (*see page 139*) or periodic limb movement (*see pages 143-44*) could be causing the problem. With these disorders your sleep can be disturbed without your being conscious of any disturbance (your partner may be able to shed some light here).

Daily questions

There is also a question that needs to be completed in the morning to help you assess the quality of your sleep. Here, you have to decide how you feel, rather than putting a cross on a scale (*see page 77*). You need to decide, on balance, if you are depressed or sleepy (wanting to go back to sleep), or tired (not sleeping, but feeling that you should feel sleepy). Circle the answer most appropriate for each question. In addition, you can mark up activities and disturbers through the night using the abbreviations, or you can add any additional comments underneath 'other' Activities and Disturbers section. For instance, you might have your sleep disrupted by external sources such as heat, noise or your partner, or by internal sources such as a low mood, illness or anxiety.

The day ruler

You fill in the day ruler just as you would the night ruler, marking on the relevant activities in the activity panel (*see ruler below*). If you have a nap during the day, make sure you mark this on in the sleep area across the top of the ruler.

Notes and medication

This section is to remind you of any events that might have affected your sleep – personal or work problems, for example – and also, any medication that you may have taken.

DAY RULER I • Date:

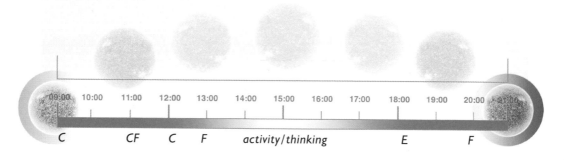

The diary

You should now be able to complete the rulers and rating scale. You need to do this for 20 days to get a good assessment of what is happening to your sleep. After 10 days, fill in the summary on pages 90–91, indicating when you went to sleep and when you woke up (*see page 126 for an example of a filled-in summary*), then go to pages 102–103 and complete the questions. You will then be able to assess your sleep and your general status. Chapter Six describes various routines and techniques that you can use to improve your sleep. In conjunction with these techniques you should then go back and complete the next 10 days of the diary. This will enable you to see if there is any improvement in your sleep. Try to fill in the diary for a typical 20-day period, not when you are on holiday or abroad on business.

If you find that you are still experiencing difficulties achieving a good night's sleep, please go to page 160 where you will find instructions on how to seek further guidance from the author's website.

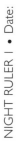

NIGHT RULER I • Date:

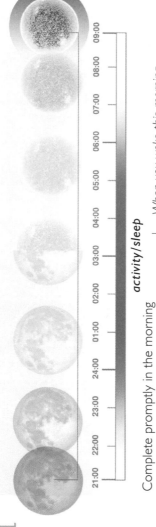

21:00 22:00 23:00 24:00 01:00 02:00 03:00 04:00 05:00 06:00 07:00 08:00 09:00

activity/sleep

Complete promptly in the morning

When you woke this morning

1. Were you depressed?	YES	NO
2. Were you sleepy?	YES	NO
3. Were you tired?	YES	NO

not refreshed/
almost unwell   OK   very
                                          refreshed

0   1   2   3   4   5   6   7   8   9   10

DAY RULER I • Date:

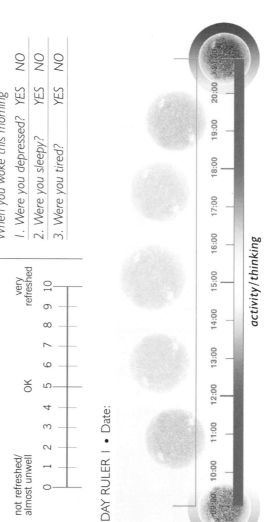

09:00 10:00 11:00 12:00 13:00 14:00 15:00 16:00 17:00 18:00 19:00 20:00 21:00

activity/thinking

Notes:

Medication:

Sleep

→	Going to bed (with the intention to sleep)
[	Lights off
↓	Going to sleep
|	Tranquil and quiet sleep
⌇	Getting up
↑	Lights on
⌐	Waking up
←	Broken, wakeful sleep

Activities and Disturbers

A Alcohol
C Caffeine
F Food
M Medicine
S Smoking
E Exercise
D Dreams
N Nightmares
I Interruption
L Lavatory
P Pain/Discomfort
W Worries
T Television/Radio
In Internet
R Reading
Other:

Sleep

→	Going to bed (with the intention to sleep)
[	Lights off
↓	Going to sleep
|	Tranquil and quiet sleep
⋀⋀	Getting up
↑	Lights on
]	Waking up
←	Broken, wakeful sleep

Activities and Disturbers

A Alcohol
C Caffeine
F Food
M Medicine
S Smoking
E Exercise
D Dreams
N Nightmares
I Interruption
L Lavatory
P Pain/Discomfort
W Worries
T Television/Radio
In Internet
R Reading
Other:

2

NIGHT RULER 2 • Date:

21:00 22:00 23:00 24:00 01:00 02:00 03:00 04:00 05:00 06:00 07:00 08:00 09:00

activity/sleep

When you woke this morning

1. Were you depressed?	YES	NO
2. Were you sleepy?	YES	NO
3. Were you tired?	YES	NO

Complete promptly in the morning

not refreshed/
almost unwell   OK   very refreshed

0   1   2   3   4   5   6   7   8   9   10

DAY RULER 2 • Date:

09:00 10:00 11:00 12:00 13:00 14:00 15:00 16:00 17:00 18:00 19:00 20:00 21:00

activity/thinking

Notes:

Medication:

3

NIGHT RULER 3 • Date:

21:00 22:00 23:00 24:00 01:00 02:00 03:00 04:00 05:00 06:00 07:00 08:00 09:00

activity/sleep

Complete promptly in the morning

When you woke this morning

1. Were you depressed?	YES	NO
2. Were you sleepy?	YES	NO
3. Were you tired?	YES	NO

not refreshed/   OK   very
almost unwell   refreshed

0   1   2   3   4   5   6   7   8   9   10

DAY RULER 3 • Date:

09:00 10:00 11:00 12:00 13:00 14:00 15:00 16:00 17:00 18:00 19:00 20:00 21:00

activity/thinking

Notes:

Medication:

Sleep

→	Going to bed (with the intention to sleep)
[	Lights off
↓	Going to sleep
|	Tranquil and quiet sleep
↑	Getting up
]	Lights on
←	Waking up
⌇	Broken, wakeful sleep

Activities and Disturbers

A Alcohol
C Caffeine
F Food
M Medicine
S Smoking
E Exercise
D Dreams
N Nightmares
I Interruption
L Lavatory
P Pain/Discomfort
W Worries
T Television/Radio
In Internet
R Reading
Other:

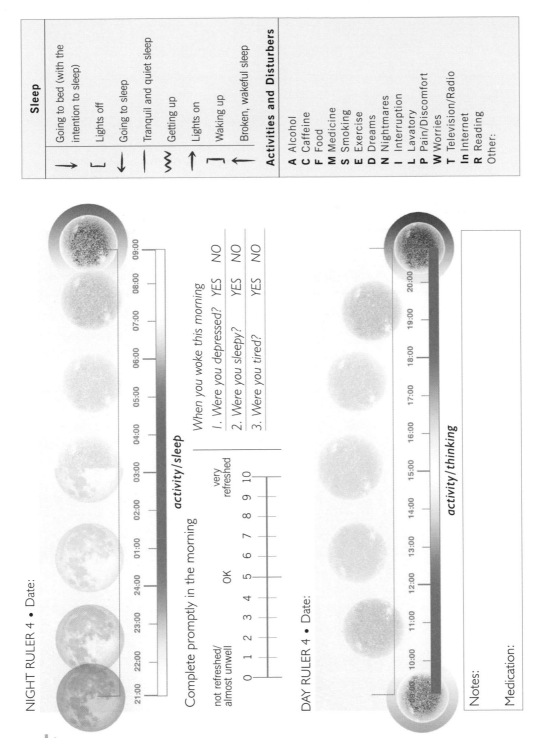

Sleep

→	Going to bed (with the intention to sleep)
[	Lights off
↓	Going to sleep
		Tranquil and quiet sleep
∿∿	Getting up
↑	Lights on
]	Waking up
←	Broken, wakeful sleep

Activities and Disturbers

A Alcohol
C Caffeine
F Food
M Medicine
S Smoking
E Exercise
D Dreams
N Nightmares
I Interruption
L Lavatory
P Pain/Discomfort
W Worries
T Television/Radio
In Internet
R Reading
Other:

4

NIGHT RULER 4 • Date:

21:00 22:00 23:00 24:00 01:00 02:00 03:00 04:00 05:00 06:00 07:00 08:00 09:00

activity/sleep

Complete promptly in the morning

When you woke this morning

1. Were you depressed? YES NO
2. Were you sleepy? YES NO
3. Were you tired? YES NO

not refreshed/almost unwell   OK   very refreshed

0 1 2 3 4 5 6 7 8 9 10

DAY RULER 4 • Date:

09:00 10:00 11:00 12:00 13:00 14:00 15:00 16:00 17:00 18:00 19:00 20:00

activity/thinking

Notes:

Medication:

5

Sleep

→	Going to bed (with the intention to sleep)
[	Lights off
↓	Going to sleep
|	Tranquil and quiet sleep
⟋	Getting up
↑	Lights on
⌐	Waking up
←	Broken, wakeful sleep

Activities and Disturbers

A Alcohol
C Caffeine
F Food
M Medicine
S Smoking
E Exercise
D Dreams
N Nightmares
I Interruption
L Lavatory
P Pain/Discomfort
W Worries
T Television/Radio
In Internet
R Reading
Other:

NIGHT RULER 5 • Date:

activity/sleep

21:00 22:00 23:00 24:00 01:00 02:00 03:00 04:00 05:00 06:00 07:00 08:00 09:00

Complete promptly in the morning

When you woke this morning

1. Were you depressed?	YES	NO
2. Were you sleepy?	YES	NO
3. Were you tired?	YES	NO

not refreshed/almost unwell   OK   very refreshed

0   1   2   3   4   5   6   7   8   9   10

DAY RULER 5 • Date:

activity/thinking

09:00 10:00 11:00 12:00 13:00 14:00 15:00 16:00 17:00 18:00 19:00 20:00 21:00

Notes:

Medication:

Sleep

→	Going to bed (with the intention to sleep)
[	Lights off
↓	Going to sleep
|	Tranquil and quiet sleep
⌇	Getting up
↑	Lights on
]	Waking up
←	Broken, wakeful sleep

Activities and Disturbers

A Alcohol
C Caffeine
F Food
M Medicine
S Smoking
E Exercise
D Dreams
N Nightmares
I Interruption
L Lavatory
P Pain/Discomfort
W Worries
T Television/Radio
In Internet
R Reading
Other:

6

NIGHT RULER 6 • Date:

21:00 22:00 23:00 24:00 01:00 02:00 03:00 04:00 05:00 06:00 07:00 08:00 09:00

activity/sleep

When you woke this morning

1. Were you depressed?   YES   NO
2. Were you sleepy?   YES   NO
3. Were you tired?   YES   NO

Complete promptly in the morning

not refreshed/   OK   very
almost unwell   refreshed

0   1   2   3   4   5   6   7   8   9   10

DAY RULER 6 • Date:

09:00 10:00 11:00 12:00 13:00 14:00 15:00 16:00 17:00 18:00 19:00 20:00

activity/thinking

Notes:

Medication:

7

NIGHT RULER 7 • Date:

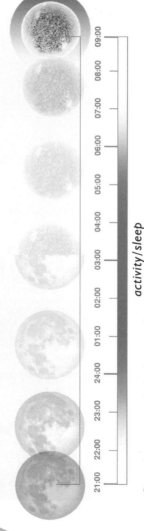

21:00	22:00	23:00	24:00	01:00	02:00	03:00	04:00	05:00	06:00	07:00	08:00	09:00

activity/sleep

Complete promptly in the morning

When you woke this morning

1. Were you depressed?	YES	NO
2. Were you sleepy?	YES	NO
3. Were you tired?	YES	NO

not refreshed/ almost unwell   OK   very refreshed

0	1	2	3	4	5	6	7	8	9	10

DAY RULER 7 • Date:

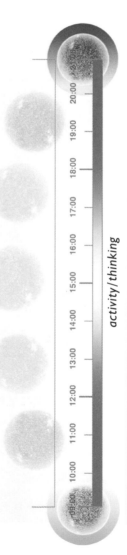

09:00	10:00	11:00	12:00	13:00	14:00	15:00	16:00	17:00	18:00	19:00	20:00

activity/thinking

Notes:

Medication:

Sleep

→	Going to bed (with the intention to sleep)
[	Lights off
↓	Going to sleep
|	Tranquil and quiet sleep
⌇	Getting up
.	Lights on
↑	Waking up
]	Broken, wakeful sleep
←	

Activities and Disturbers

A Alcohol
C Caffeine
F Food
M Medicine
S Smoking
E Exercise
D Dreams
N Nightmares
I Interruption
L Lavatory
P Pain/Discomfort
W Worries
T Television/Radio
In Internet
R Reading
Other:

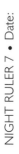

Sleep

→	Going to bed (with the intention to sleep)
[	Lights off
↓	Going to sleep
|	Tranquil and quiet sleep
⌇	Getting up
↑	Lights on
⌐	Waking up
←	Broken, wakeful sleep

Activities and Disturbers

A Alcohol
C Caffeine
F Food
M Medicine
S Smoking
E Exercise
D Dreams
N Nightmares
I Interruption
L Lavatory
P Pain/Discomfort
W Worries
T Television/Radio
In Internet
R Reading
Other:

8

NIGHT RULER 8 • Date:

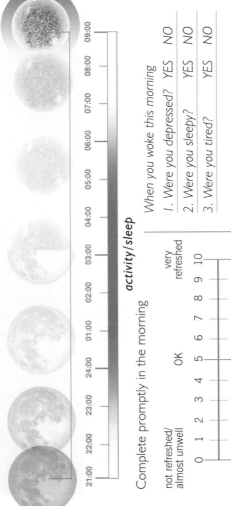

21:00 22:00 23:00 24:00 01:00 02:00 03:00 04:00 05:00 06:00 07:00 08:00 09:00

activity/sleep

Complete promptly in the morning

When you woke this morning

1. Were you depressed?	YES	NO
2. Were you sleepy?	YES	NO
3. Were you tired?	YES	NO

not refreshed/
almost unwell   OK   very
                                          refreshed

0   1   2   3   4   5   6   7   8   9   10

DAY RULER 8 • Date:

09:00 10:00 11:00 12:00 13:00 14:00 15:00 16:00 17:00 18:00 19:00 20:00 21:00

activity/thinking

Notes:

Medication:

Sleep

→	Going to bed (with the intention to sleep)
[	Lights off
↓	Going to sleep
|	Tranquil and quiet sleep
⌇	
↑	Getting up
⌐	Lights on
←	Waking up
	Broken, wakeful sleep

Activities and Disturbers

A Alcohol
C Caffeine
F Food
M Medicine
S Smoking
E Exercise
D Dreams
N Nightmares
I Interruption
L Lavatory
P Pain/Discomfort
W Worries
T Television/Radio
In Internet
R Reading
Other:

9

NIGHT RULER 9 • Date:

21:00 22:00 23:00 24:00 01:00 02:00 03:00 04:00 05:00 06:00 07:00 08:00 09:00

activity/sleep

Complete promptly in the morning

When you woke this morning

1. Were you depressed? YES   NO
2. Were you sleepy?   YES   NO
3. Were you tired?   YES   NO

not refreshed/almost unwell   OK   very refreshed

0   1   2   3   4   5   6   7   8   9   10

DAY RULER 9 • Date:

09:00 10:00 11:00 12:00 13:00 14:00 15:00 16:00 17:00 18:00 19:00 20:00 21:00

activity/thinking

Notes:

Medication:

Sleep

→	Going to bed (with the intention to sleep)
[	Lights off
↓	Going to sleep
|	Tranquil and quiet sleep
∿	Getting up
]	Lights on
↑	Waking up
←	Broken, wakeful sleep

Activities and Disturbers

A Alcohol
C Caffeine
F Food
M Medicine
S Smoking
E Exercise
D Dreams
N Nightmares
I Interruption
L Lavatory
P Pain/Discomfort
W Worries
T Television/Radio
In Internet
R Reading
Other:

10

NIGHT RULER 10 • Date:

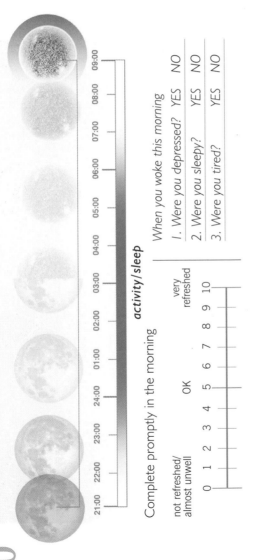

21:00 22:00 23:00 24:00 01:00 02:00 03:00 04:00 05:00 06:00 07:00 08:00 09:00

activity/sleep

Complete promptly in the morning

When you woke this morning

1. Were you depressed?	YES	NO
2. Were you sleepy?	YES	NO
3. Were you tired?	YES	NO

not refreshed/almost unwell   OK   very refreshed

0 1 2 3 4 5 6 7 8 9 10

DAY RULER 10 • Date:

09:00 10:00 11:00 12:00 13:00 14:00 15:00 16:00 17:00 18:00 19:00 20:00

activity/thinking

Notes:

Medication:

Summary

NIGHT RULER 1 • Date:

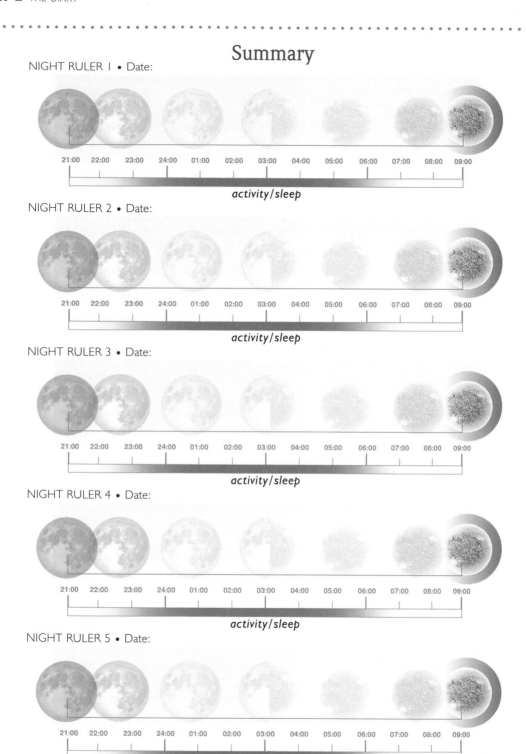

NIGHT RULER 2 • Date:

NIGHT RULER 3 • Date:

NIGHT RULER 4 • Date:

NIGHT RULER 5 • Date:

NIGHT RULER 6 • Date:

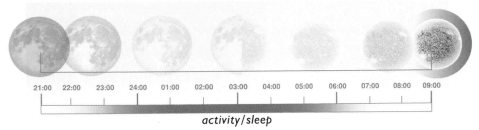

activity/sleep

NIGHT RULER 7 • Date:

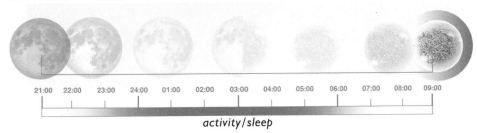

activity/sleep

NIGHT RULER 8 • Date:

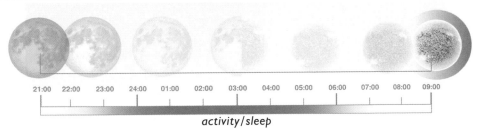

activity/sleep

NIGHT RULER 9 • Date:

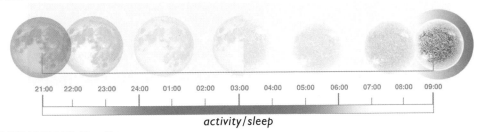

activity/sleep

NIGHT RULER 10 • Date:

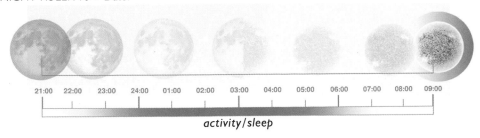

activity/sleep

Sleep

→	Going to bed (with the intention to sleep)
[	Lights off
↓	Going to sleep
∿	Tranquil and quiet sleep
↑	Getting up
]	Lights on
←	Waking up
	Broken, wakeful sleep

Activities and Disturbers

A Alcohol
C Caffeine
F Food
M Medicine
S Smoking
E Exercise
D Dreams
N Nightmares
I Interruption
L Lavatory
P Pain/Discomfort
W Worries
T Television/Radio
In Internet
R Reading
Other:

11

NIGHT RULER 11 • Date:

21:00 22:00 23:00 24:00 01:00 02:00 03:00 04:00 05:00 06:00 07:00 08:00 09:00

activity/sleep

When you woke this morning

1. Were you depressed?   YES   NO
2. Were you sleepy?   YES   NO
3. Were you tired?   YES   NO

Complete promptly in the morning

not refreshed/   OK   very
almost unwell   refreshed

0   1   2   3   4   5   6   7   8   9   10

DAY RULER 11 • Date:

09:00 10:00 11:00 12:00 13:00 14:00 15:00 16:00 17:00 18:00 19:00 20:00 21:00

activity/thinking

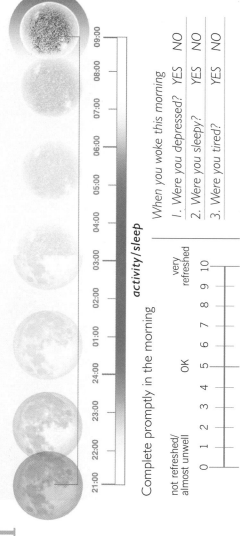

Notes:

Medication:

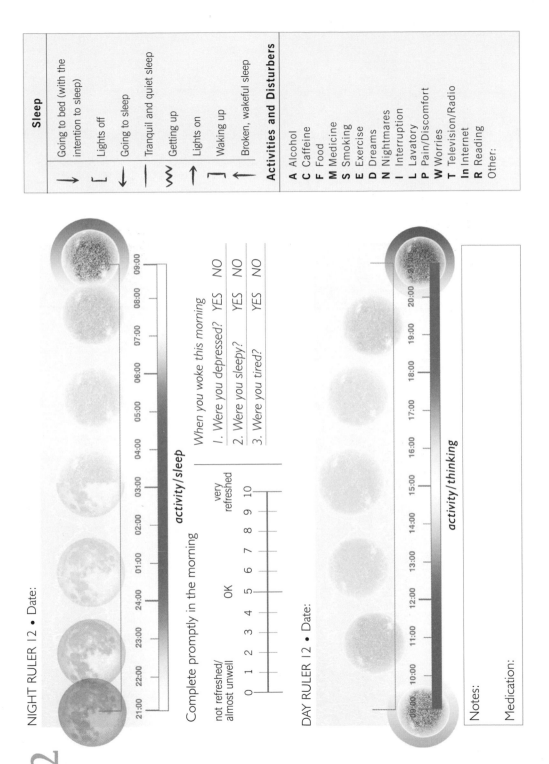

12

NIGHT RULER 12 • Date:

21:00 22:00 23:00 24:00 01:00 02:00 03:00 04:00 05:00 06:00 07:00 08:00 09:00

activity/sleep

Complete promptly in the morning

not refreshed/
almost unwell   OK   very
                                             refreshed

0   1   2   3   4   5   6   7   8   9   10

When you woke this morning

1. Were you depressed?   YES   NO
2. Were you sleepy?   YES   NO
3. Were you tired?   YES   NO

DAY RULER 12 • Date:

09:00 10:00 11:00 12:00 13:00 14:00 15:00 16:00 17:00 18:00 19:00 20:00 21:00

activity/thinking

Notes:

Medication:

Sleep

→   Going to bed (with the intention to sleep)

[Lights off

↓   Going to sleep

| Tranquil and quiet sleep

∿   Getting up

↑   Lights on

]   Waking up

←   Broken, wakeful sleep

Activities and Disturbers

A Alcohol
C Caffeine
F Food
M Medicine
S Smoking
E Exercise
D Dreams
N Nightmares
I Interruption
L Lavatory
P Pain/Discomfort
W Worries
T Television/Radio
In Internet
R Reading
Other:

Sleep	
→	Going to bed (with the intention to sleep)
[	Lights off
↓	Going to sleep
|\\\\	Tranquil and quiet sleep
↑	Getting up
]	Lights on
←	Waking up
	Broken, wakeful sleep

Activities and Disturbers

A Alcohol
C Caffeine
F Food
M Medicine
S Smoking
E Exercise
D Dreams
N Nightmares
I Interruption
L Lavatory
P Pain/Discomfort
W Worries
T Television/Radio
In Internet
R Reading
Other:

13

NIGHT RULER 13 • Date:

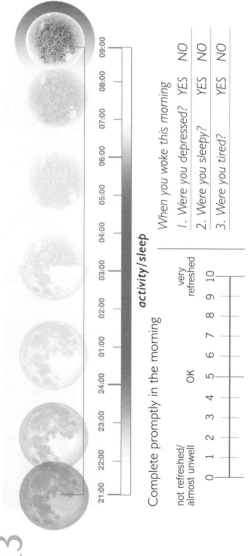

21:00 22:00 23:00 24:00 01:00 02:00 03:00 04:00 05:00 06:00 07:00 08:00 09:00

activity/sleep

Complete promptly in the morning

not refreshed/
almost unwell   OK   very
                                         refreshed

0   1   2   3   4   5   6   7   8   9   10

When you woke this morning

1. Were you depressed?	YES	NO
2. Were you sleepy?	YES	NO
3. Were you tired?	YES	NO

DAY RULER 13 • Date:

09:00 10:00 11:00 12:00 13:00 14:00 15:00 16:00 17:00 18:00 19:00 20:00

activity/thinking

Notes:

Medication:

14

NIGHT RULER 14 • Date:

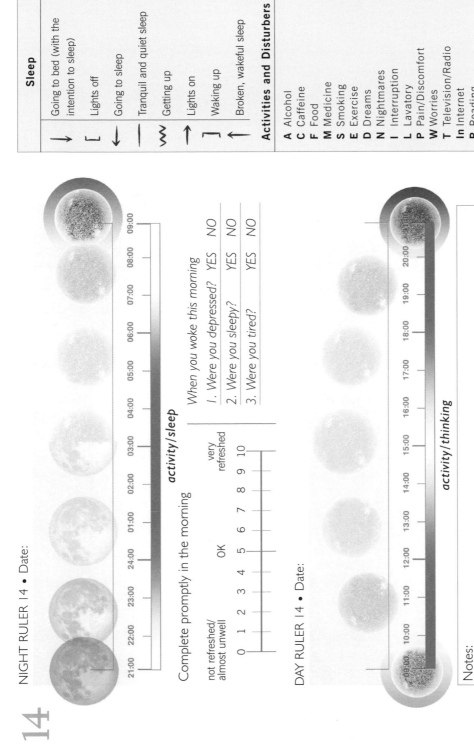

Sleep	
→	Going to bed (with the intention to sleep)
[	Lights off
↓	Going to sleep
|	Tranquil and quiet sleep
∿	Getting up
↑	Lights on
⌐	Waking up
←	Broken, wakeful sleep

Activities and Disturbers

A Alcohol
C Caffeine
F Food
M Medicine
S Smoking
E Exercise
D Dreams
N Nightmares
I Interruption
L Lavatory
P Pain/Discomfort
W Worries
T Television/Radio
In Internet
R Reading
Other:

21:00 22:00 23:00 24:00 01:00 02:00 03:00 04:00 05:00 06:00 07:00 08:00 09:00

activity/sleep

Complete promptly in the morning

When you woke this morning

1. Were you depressed?	YES	NO
2. Were you sleepy?	YES	NO
3. Were you tired?	YES	NO

not refreshed/   OK   very
almost unwell   refreshed

0 1 2 3 4 5 6 7 8 9 10

DAY RULER 14 • Date:

09:00 10:00 11:00 12:00 13:00 14:00 15:00 16:00 17:00 18:00 19:00 20:00

activity/thinking

Notes:

Medication:

15

NIGHT RULER 15 • Date:

21:00 22:00 23:00 24:00 01:00 02:00 03:00 04:00 05:00 06:00 07:00 08:00 09:00

activity / sleep

Complete promptly in the morning

not refreshed/ almost unwell				OK					very refreshed	
0	1	2	3	4	5	6	7	8	9	10

When you woke this morning

1. Were you depressed?	YES	NO
2. Were you sleepy?	YES	NO
3. Were you tired?	YES	NO

DAY RULER 15 • Date:

09:00 10:00 11:00 12:00 13:00 14:00 15:00 16:00 17:00 18:00 19:00 20:00 21:00

activity / thinking

Notes:

Medication:

Sleep

→	Going to bed (with the intention to sleep)
[	Lights off
↓	Going to sleep
⋙	Tranquil and quiet sleep
		Getting up
↑	Lights on
]	Waking up
←	Broken, wakeful sleep

Activities and Disturbers

A Alcohol
C Caffeine
F Food
M Medicine
S Smoking
E Exercise
D Dreams
N Nightmares
I Interruption
L Lavatory
P Pain/Discomfort
W Worries
T Television/Radio
In Internet
R Reading
Other:

16

NIGHT RULER 16 • Date:

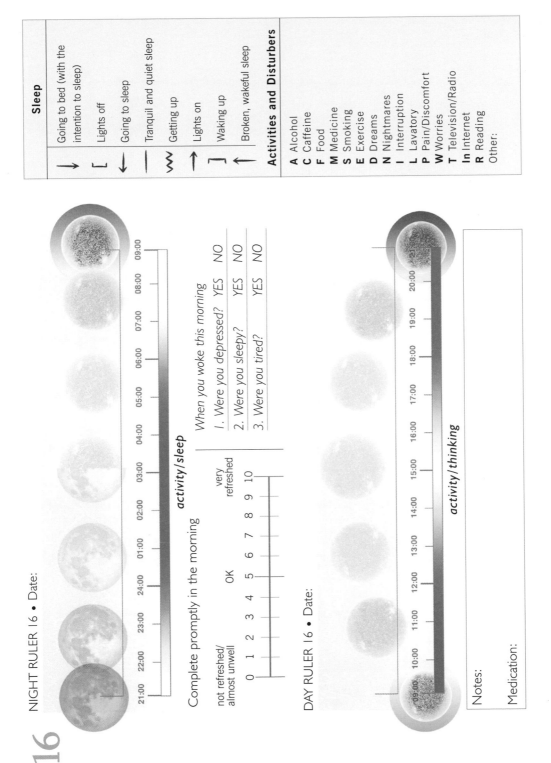

Sleep

→	Going to bed (with the intention to sleep)
[	Lights off
↓	Going to sleep
|	Tranquil and quiet sleep
∿	Getting up
↑	Lights on
⌐	Waking up
←	Broken, wakeful sleep

Activities and Disturbers

A Alcohol
C Caffeine
F Food
M Medicine
S Smoking
E Exercise
D Dreams
N Nightmares
I Interruption
L Lavatory
P Pain/Discomfort
W Worries
T Television/Radio
In Internet
R Reading
Other:

21:00 22:00 23:00 24:00 01:00 02:00 03:00 04:00 05:00 06:00 07:00 08:00 09:00

activity/sleep

Complete promptly in the morning

When you woke this morning

1. Were you depressed?	YES	NO
2. Were you sleepy?	YES	NO
3. Were you tired?	YES	NO

not refreshed/ almost unwell   OK   very refreshed

0 1 2 3 4 5 6 7 8 9 10

DAY RULER 16 • Date:

09:00 10:00 11:00 12:00 13:00 14:00 15:00 16:00 17:00 18:00 19:00 20:00 21:00

activity/thinking

Notes:

Medication:

17

NIGHT RULER 17 • Date:

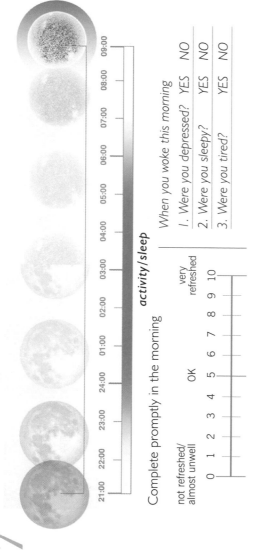

21:00 22:00 23:00 24:00 01:00 02:00 03:00 04:00 05:00 06:00 07:00 08:00 09:00

activity/sleep

Complete promptly in the morning

not refreshed/ almost unwell					OK					very refreshed
0	1	2	3	4	5	6	7	8	9	10

When you woke this morning

1. Were you depressed?   YES   NO
2. Were you sleepy?   YES   NO
3. Were you tired?   YES   NO

DAY RULER 17 • Date:

09:00 10:00 11:00 12:00 13:00 14:00 15:00 16:00 17:00 18:00 19:00 20:00 21:00

activity/thinking

Notes:

Medication:

Sleep

→	Going to bed (with the intention to sleep)
[	Lights off
↓	Going to sleep
│	Tranquil and quiet sleep
〰	Getting up
↑	Lights on
]	Waking up
←	Broken, wakeful sleep

Activities and Disturbers

A Alcohol
C Caffeine
F Food
M Medicine
S Smoking
E Exercise
D Dreams
N Nightmares
I Interruption
L Lavatory
P Pain/Discomfort
W Worries
T Television/Radio
In Internet
R Reading
Other:

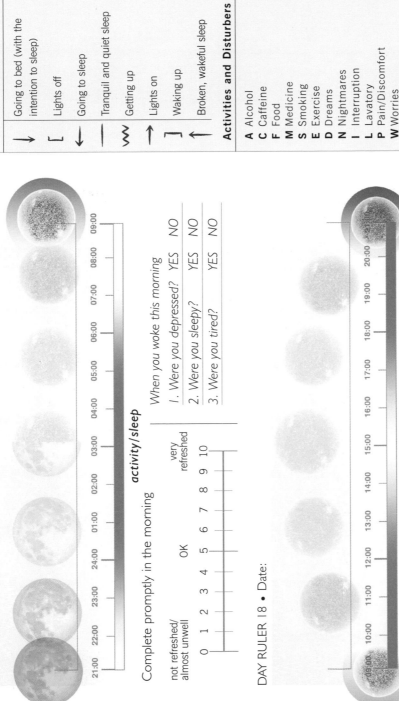

Sleep

→	Going to bed (with the intention to sleep)
[	Lights off
↓	Going to sleep
〰	Tranquil and quiet sleep
↑	Getting up
]	Lights on
←	Waking up
	Broken, wakeful sleep

Activities and Disturbers

A Alcohol
C Caffeine
F Food
M Medicine
S Smoking
E Exercise
D Dreams
N Nightmares
I Interruption
L Lavatory
P Pain/Discomfort
W Worries
T Television/Radio
In Internet
R Reading
Other:

18

NIGHT RULER 18 • Date:

21:00 22:00 23:00 24:00 01:00 02:00 03:00 04:00 05:00 06:00 07:00 08:00 09:00

activity/sleep

Complete promptly in the morning

When you woke this morning

1. Were you depressed?	YES	NO
2. Were you sleepy?	YES	NO
3. Were you tired?	YES	NO

not refreshed/almost unwell   OK   very refreshed

0 1 2 3 4 5 6 7 8 9 10

DAY RULER 18 • Date:

09:00 10:00 11:00 12:00 13:00 14:00 15:00 16:00 17:00 18:00 19:00 20:00 21:00

activity/thinking

Notes:

Medication:

19

NIGHT RULER 19 • Date:

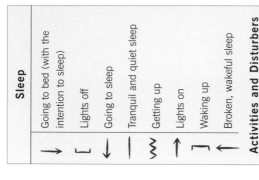

21:00 22:00 23:00 24:00 01:00 02:00 03:00 04:00 05:00 06:00 07:00 08:00 09:00

activity/sleep

Complete promptly in the morning

When you woke this morning

1. Were you depressed? YES NO
2. Were you sleepy? YES NO
3. Were you tired? YES NO

not refreshed/
almost unwell   OK   very
refreshed

0 1 2 3 4 5 6 7 8 9 10

DAY RULER 19 • Date:

09:00 10:00 11:00 12:00 13:00 14:00 15:00 16:00 17:00 18:00 19:00 20:00 21:00

activity/thinking

Notes:

Medication:

Sleep

→	Going to bed (with the intention to sleep)
[	Lights off
↓	Going to sleep
/	Tranquil and quiet sleep
∿	Getting up
↑	Lights on
⌐	Waking up
←	Broken, wakeful sleep

Activities and Disturbers

A Alcohol
C Caffeine
F Food
M Medicine
S Smoking
E Exercise
D Dreams
N Nightmares
I Interruption
L Lavatory
P Pain/Discomfort
W Worries
T Television/Radio
In Internet
R Reading
Other:

Sleep

→	Going to bed (with the intention to sleep)
[	Lights off
↓	Going to sleep
|	Tranquil and quiet sleep
∿	Broken, wakeful sleep
↑	Getting up
]	Lights on
←	Waking up

Activities and Disturbers

A Alcohol
C Caffeine
F Food
M Medicine
S Smoking
E Exercise
D Dreams
N Nightmares
I Interruption
L Lavatory
P Pain/Discomfort
W Worries
T Television/Radio
In Internet
R Reading
Other:

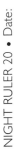

NIGHT RULER 20 • Date:

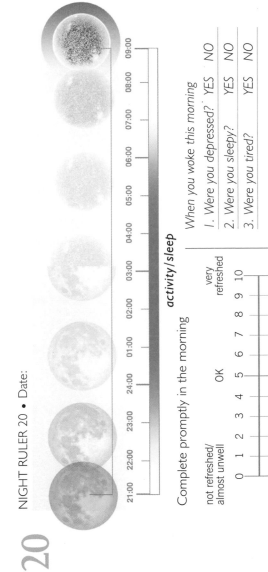

21:00 22:00 23:00 24:00 01:00 02:00 03:00 04:00 05:00 06:00 07:00 08:00 09:00

activity/sleep

Complete promptly in the morning

When you woke this morning

1. Were you depressed?	YES	NO
2. Were you sleepy?	YES	NO
3. Were you tired?	YES	NO

not refreshed/
almost unwell   OK   very refreshed

0 1 2 3 4 5 6 7 8 9 10

DAY RULER 20 • Date:

09:00 10:00 11:00 12:00 13:00 14:00 15:00 16:00 17:00 18:00 19:00 20:00

activity/thinking

Notes:

Medication:

The questions

The questions on the following pages do not by themselves provide a definitive assess-ment of character, mood or the cause of the sleep disorder, but they do offer clues. These are not quantitative tools, but qualitative. Definitive assessments should be obtained through professional services, but this book may provide the answers that will allow you to help yourself. The questions give you a framework against which to assess the results from your day and night rulers, ratings scales and daily questions. It is worthwhile com-pleting these questions early on in your assessment in case you find that you are scoring high on a measure such as anxiety or alcoholism. If this is the case then you might want to seek help for this. Completing the sleep diaries and then following the instructions on how to improve your sleep should strengthen your sleep, even though they do not tackle your core difficulty. These questions ask for 'yes' or 'no' responses (tick the relevant column). 'Don't know' is not an option. The appraisals are found on pages 106–07.

Depressed mood	Yes	No
I am bothered by things that used not to bother me		
I think my life has been a failure		
I am not happy most of the time		
I don't socialize as much as I used to		
I feel lonely		
I don't enjoy life		
I feel sad		
I am depressed most of the time		
I can't concentrate on anything		
Anxiety		
I am usually apprehensive		
I can't relax easily		
I suffer from tense muscles		
My mouth is often dry		
I suffer from diarrhoea quite often		
I often sweat a lot during the day		
I often feel on edge		
I often get butterflies in my stomach		
I am often anxious		
Alcoholism		
Have you ever had a problem with alcohol?		
Have you ever been told by friends that you have a problem with alcohol?		
Have you ever been told by friends or relatives that you drink too much alcohol?		
Do you consume more than three alcoholic drinks in the evening?		
Do you drink alcohol before bedtime to put yourself to sleep?		

Worry-centred insomnia	Yes	No
I worry before I go to bed that I will sleep badly		
If I wake up in the middle of the night, I worry about getting back to sleep		
My mind keeps turning things over		
My thinking takes a long time to 'unwind'		
Often when I am half-asleep I am still trying to follow the train of my thoughts		
I cannot empty my mind before going to sleep		
Tense insomnia		
I find it hard to let go		
My body is full of tension		
I find it difficult to physically relax my body		
I suffer from tension headaches		
My muscles ache all the time		
My back is often painful		
Stimulus-control insomnia		
When I get into bed I often feel more awake		
I spend time reading/watching TV		
I sleep better when I am not in my own bed		
I often fall asleep in the living room		
Insomnia-related		
I know I won't sleep well		
I can't concentrate unless I have slept well		
A bad night's sleep leaves me exhausted the next day		
I feel dissatisfied with the depth of my sleep		
I can't cope unless I have slept well		
I know I will feel unwell if I don't sleep properly		
I look awful if I haven't slept properly		

Biological clock: phase advance	Yes	No
I tire quickly in the evening		
I keep going to bed earlier and earlier		
I can't get my sleep into a proper routine		
I can't control my sleep		
I don't understand why my bedtime seems to be getting earlier and earlier		
Biological clock: phase delay		
I don't feel tired enough at bedtime		
My bedtime gets later during the week		
I can't wake up when I want to		
My brain doesn't function until lunch-time		
I keep going to bed later and later		
Medicines: sleeping pills		
Have you taken medicines for your nerves recently?		
Do you have to take more pills to feel any effect?		
Have you ever been prescribed medicines for sleep?		
Do you have problems stopping taking sleeping pills?		
Drugs: social abuse		
Do you take drugs regularly?		
Have you ever taken illegal drugs?		
If you consume illegal drugs is it recreational or does your life revolve around them?		
Have you consumed illegal drugs recently?		

Appraisals

If you have answered yes to three or more questions in any section, reconsider how you have filled in the questionnaire and how long you have been feeling this way and follow the advice given below.

Depressed mood

If you have previously been treated for depression, then you may score higher on this table. If your current mood is poor then consider seeking further help. Depression is often associated with early-morning awakening and some phase-advance of the sleep-awake cycle.

Anxiety

If you have previously been treated for anxiety then you should consider and act on the advice and treatment that has been effective before. Try the relaxation exercises included in this book (*see pages 120–26*).

Alcoholism

If you have been treated for alcoholism then continue with the other sections and consider how to strengthen your sleep. Sleep studies indicate that it may take a year or longer for sleep to recover from chronic alcoholism.

Worry-centred insomnia

Are you a worrier? Worry can increase the state of alertness. You might consider tackling worry directly as well as using the exercises that may displace your worries (*see pages 123–26*). You should also double-check the biological clock questions. It is possible that you are being woken up by this (and possibly other causes such as pain, needing to go to the lavatory and so on) and because you are awake, you are spending your time worrying.

Tense insomnia

If, on balance, you feel that tension is a significant factor then you should certainly use the progressive muscular relaxation exercise (*see pages 122–23*). You might also consider the responses under 'sleep-centred insomnia' as worry can lead to tension.

Stimulus-control insomnia

If, on the whole, you agree with the overall direction of the questions asked, you may have conditioned yourself to remaining awake in bed as opposed to sleeping. The chances are that other factors are involved, but if your insomnia started with a significant life event such as bereavement and you had slept well before, plus, there is no medical history that might explain the sleeplessness, then it is possible that sleep-lessness caused by the life event has turned into an insomnia. There is a specific way of tackling this: Bootzin Stimulus Control (*see page 120*).

Insomnia-related

If, on balance, this describes you, then refer to the section on inappropriate sleep-inducing behaviours and beliefs (*see page 127*). It is likely that you will have scored highly on one or more of the other insomnia tables as well, so you could try some of the suggestions associated with those tables. Finally, if all else fails, you should go back and review Chapters One, Two and Three.

Biological clock: phase advance

If, on balance, this describes you, then you may be suffering from a biological clock that is running too quickly. See the section on circadian disorders and phase advance in particular (*see page 144*).

Biological clock: phase delay

If, on balance, this describes you, then your biological clock may be running too slowly. See the section on circadian disorders and phase delay in particular (*see pages 144–45*).

Drugs and medicines

If, on balance, this describes you, it suggests that you have developed an insomnia syndrome. You will probably have scored highly in some of the other tables, so apply the solutions you find there. Also, read the section on sleeping pills (*see pages 114–16*). Chronic insomniacs often find themselves on a cycle of misuse of hypnotics and inadvertently perpetuate their problems. Is caffeine the problem (*see pages 48–9*)?

So many medicines affect sleep that it is surprising there are not more problems. Clearly, the advice for drugs of abuse and social drugs is to control their intake (you need specialist advice for this). In the case of conventional medicines, you should go back to Chapters One and Two and work out how to strengthen your own sleep system to overcome the disturbing effects of your medication.

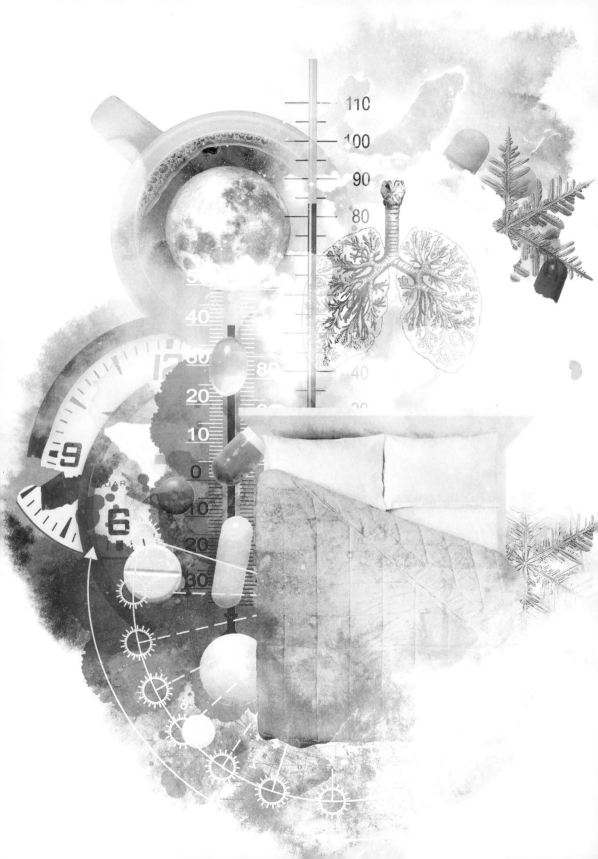

CHAPTER SIX

Dealing with disturbed sleep

. . . .

This chapter helps you to evaluate what you have learned from the diary and questionnaires and helps you to decide whether you are suffering from true insomnia or some other sleep disorder. It suggests some exercises that can help promote sleep.

The diagram below illustrates many of the ideas introduced in the earlier chapters. Its purpose is to help you understand why some therapeutic strategies work and some do not. The main points are:

- Some people react to stress by tensing their muscles. Increased muscle tension increases pressure from the awake system that prevents sleep from taking place.
- Other people have medical problems that produce muscle rigidity and this has the same effect of preventing sleep.
- Some may have worries that partially activate the fight/flight systems. These also promote activity in the awake system and so prevent sleep.
- Intrusive thoughts and emotional imagery may activate the arousal systems and/or increase muscle tension, resulting in increased activity in the awake system. Finally, the biological clock may influence either sleep onset time or waking up time. This depends on heredity, as well as early learning and subsequent conditioning. If the clock is the problem and is alerting the awake system, then the effectiveness of sleep-control techniques such as muscle relaxation, abdominal breathing, meditation and so on will be limited. It is possible to change your clock, using light. See the section on jet lag (*see pages 58–9*).

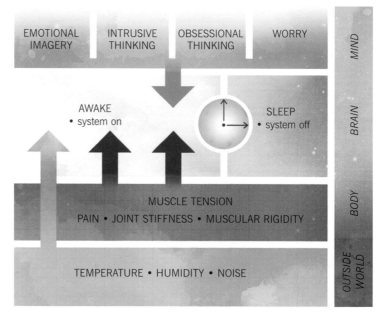

There are various factors that can stop you sleeping by increasing activity in the awake system. The exercises and techniques included in this chapter show you how to deal with their input, thus allowing you to go to sleep.

Examining the diary rulers

You will now have filled in the diary. The first thing to do is to calculate the average amount of time you spend asleep every 24 hours (including naps and times of troubled or light sleep). While you are doing this, see whether there are any consistent patterns to your sleep. The purpose of working out your average amount of sleep is to provide a baseline from which to work on and improve.

- Are there any consistent patterns? Ask yourself the following questions:
- Are weekends having an effect on my sleep?
- How much caffeine do I consume (*see pages 48–9*)?
- How much alcohol do I drink (*see pages 49–50*)?
- How many cigarettes do I smoke (*see page 50*)?
- Are soft drugs affecting my sleep (*see pages 52–3*)?
- Is sex a problem? Should I discuss it with my partner?

Start by looking for the obvious and if that doesn't lead anywhere then consider whether it is a combination of factors that is causing the problem. Remember that one disturbed night will also affect the next and sometimes even the following night. This will happen even if the sleep, awake and clock systems are all operating normally.

Are most nights the same? For chronic insomniacs the nights are often different. This inconsistency is regarded by some as the hallmark of insomnia.

Frequent patterns: individual nights

If your night-time rulers generally look like one of the two shown on the next page and you wake up quickly, feel refreshed and don't feel you have a problem – then you don't! Short sleepers tend to have less light sleep (stage 2) than average or long sleepers and conversely, long sleepers tend to have more light sleep. As this stage appears to act simply as a 'filler', having more or less of it is probably not important. Short sleepers can enjoy the extra time awake to pursue other activities. Long sleepers should simply enjoy their long stay in bed. If long sleepers need to remain awake, they must remember that the pressure for sleep will remain and so they should be vigilant if they are involved in monotonous work. Other variations of normal sleep are illustrated in Chapter Three.

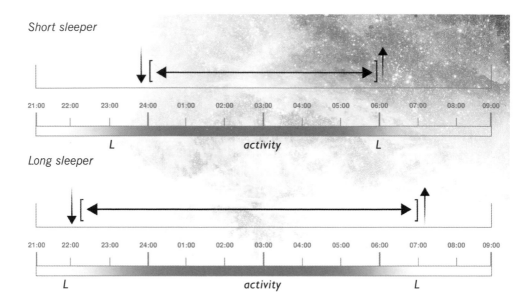

Unrefreshing sleep

If your sleep seems sound, but you consistently wake up unrefreshed and feel tired and sleepy during the day – or if you find that you fall asleep easily on buses, trains, watching TV and so on – then you might be suffering from a disorder that is disturbing your sleep, but not sufficiently to wake you up. The cause might be your bed. Your bed is certainly suspect if you suffer from aches and pains for the first few hours after getting up and subsequently feel better. The wrong sheets, pillows or duvets, uncomfortable bedroom temperature, humidity and so on may all cause these problems.

Talking to your bed-partner might help identify what is going on. If you are snoring or occasionally hold your breath, you should go to the section on snoring and sleep apnoea (*see pages 139–40*). If you move your legs around a lot during the night then you should read about periodic limb movement disorder (*see pages 143–44*).

Sleep onset problems

If your ruler looks like the one opposite you have a sleep onset problem. Do you have any routines that help to settle you before going to bed? (*see page 46*). Do you drink any beverages that contain caffeine in the evening? Do you exercise shortly before going to bed? If the problem occurs just on Sundays, read the section on weekend effect (*see pages 113–15*) and try to maintain a more regular schedule. The ruler also shows more than one hour in bed without trying to sleep. This can weaken the association between bed and sleeping. Follow the instructions for 'stimulus control' (*see page 120*).

Sleep onset problem

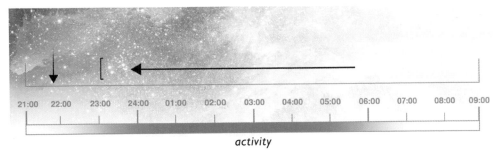

Early-morning awakening

Are you a short sleeper who is going to bed too early? Are you or have you been depressed (*see questionnaire, page 103*)? Follow the stimulus control instructions (*see page 120*) to prevent a negative association developing between bed and sleep. Depression is associated with disrupted sleep, but curiously, sleep deprivation can also relieve depression, particularly in those who are most depressed in the morning and whose depression lifts during the day. Depression may speed up the biological clock, which also leads to early-morning wakening. Exposure to evening light (or bright artificial light) may help slow the clock down and enable you to sleep longer in the morning. Do note, however, that the duration of sleep also decreases with age.

Early-morning awakening

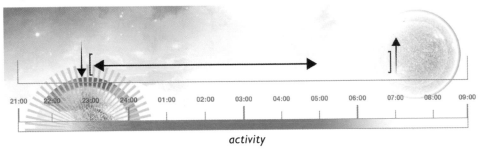

Frequent patterns: several nights

Page 115 illustrates the weekend effect, when small changes in your routine are sufficient to disrupt your sleep. Friday night shows a slightly later night than usual with just one nightcap (A). Waking up on Saturday morning is approximately 2 hours later than this person's usual weekday time. This increase reflects a sleep debt that has probably accumulated during the week.

The various activities on Saturday are omitted, although an exercise session is noted after lunch. Saturday evening involves more alcohol consumption than usual and a much later bedtime. Sleep onset is rapid but sleep is broken in the morning, partly because of the rebound effect of alcohol, also the need to go to the lavatory, which is also caused by the alcohol, and because of the biological clock. Nevertheless, broken sleep is achieved until mid-morning.

The disrupted nature of the night's sleep, and sleep occurring at a different clock time, leads to a sleep need that is partly dissipated by a mid-afternoon nap (which lessens sleep need the following evening).

Sunday night starts off with a habitual bedtime but the late mornings have probably caused a slight shift in the biological clock, which prevents sleep taking place rapidly. Once sleep does begin it is less stable than usual and ends with the Monday morning alarm call. The week starts with a tired and depressed groan. Sound familiar?

This example contained a celebratory amount of alcohol on the Saturday night, but even without the alcohol, some people may find that their change in sleep pattern during the weekend is sufficient to disrupt their sleep at the beginning of the working week. Seasonal daylight savings can produce measurable changes with a shift of only one hour.

The Sunday daytime nap is less of a problem for someone who is always striving to reduce a chronic sleep debt. An afternoon nap is unlikely to affect the biological clock, has the benefit of increasing alertness during the rest of the waking day and is unlikely to reduce the pressure for sleep during the night.

Occasional use of sleeping pills

The sequence of night rulers on page 117 illustrates what happens to someone who occasionally takes sleeping pills that have been prescribed by a medical practitioner. Most regulatory prescribing bodies recommend only short courses of sleeping pills. The value of this recommendation is not debated here. What is illustrated is someone with chronic insomnia who is trying to manage on a reduced intake of sleeping pills.

On night 1, he falls asleep quickly without a pill, but wakes up to go to the lavatory. On returning to bed, he finds his sleep is disturbed, so he takes half a sleeping pill! This is very wrong (but in my experience happens surprisingly often). First, most – although not all – sleeping pills are designed to maintain sleep throughout the night. Taking a pill halfway through the night almost certainly means that there will be a hangover effect the next day.

Hangover effects are not only unpleasant but can be dangerous, because of reduced alertness. Secondly, the dosage is calculated carefully to induce sleep quickly and main-tain that sleep. Taking half a pill may not induce sleep, and may not maintain it, but it

The Weekend Effect

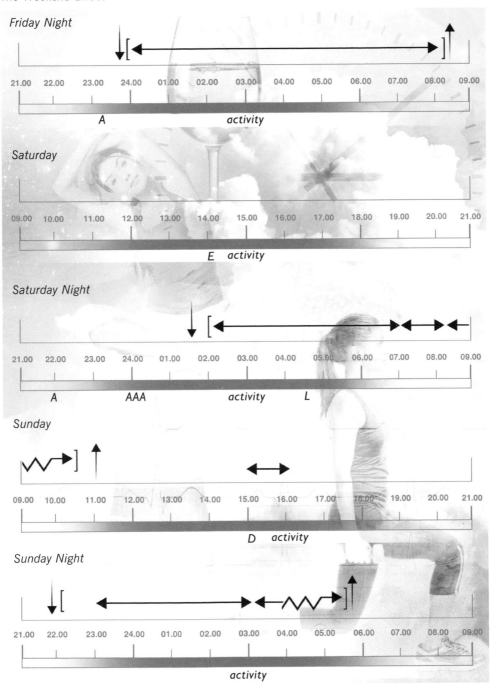

Friday Night

21.00 22.00 23.00 24.00 01.00 02.00 03.00 04.00 05.00 06.00 07.00 08.00 09.00

A   *activity*

Saturday

09.00 10.00 11.00 12.00 13.00 14.00 15.00 16.00 17.00 18.00 19.00 20.00 21.00

E *activity*

Saturday Night

21.00 22.00 23.00 24.00 01.00 02.00 03.00 04.00 05.00 06.00 07.00 08.00 09.00

A   AAA   *activity*   L

Sunday

09.00 10.00 11.00 12.00 13.00 14.00 15.00 16.00 17.00 18.00 19.00 20.00 21.00

D *activity*

Sunday Night

21.00 22.00 23.00 24.00 01.00 02.00 03.00 04.00 05.00 06.00 07.00 08.00 09.00

activity

can have sufficient strength to produce a hangover! Many chronic insomniacs become tolerant to their sleeping pills and so they increase the dose. For others who have become tolerant, the ritual of taking the pill is enough to put them back to sleep. In the situation illustrated here, it is likely that the effect of the drug is as much psychological as it is pharmacological.

Night 2 is almost a guilt night. Listening to the doctor's instructions, and feeling guilty about having taken a sleeping pill the night before, the insomniac has a night of broken sleep. One of the reasons is the sleeping pill taken the night before – rebound wakefulness (*see page 52*). On the third night, the insomniac gives in and takes a sleeping pill. It's not a great night's sleep but there is more of it than before. Unfortunately, on the fourth night, rebound wakefulness and the reduced sleep-need combine to give the insomniac a rough night's sleep.

The insomniac perseveres without a pill on night 5, and although his sleep is broken, there can be more of it. Some sleeping pills have an impact on sleep two nights afterwards, so insomniacs may have a poor night even on this night. On night 6, the insomniac again takes a pill and the 2–3 night cycle restarts. This shows that for some people intermittent use of sleeping pills may prolong insomnia.

Your doctor should give you advice on how to use sleeping pills properly. Generally, the advice is not to remain on sleeping pills for extended periods. Taking short courses (from a few days to 1–2 weeks) is straightforward, bearing in mind that the majority will cause temporary rebound wakefulness when you stop. Intermittent use is more complex, because of the possibility of rebound effects as shown opposite, both for physiological reasons (the sleep and awake systems) and pharmacological reasons (the brain responding to the absence of the sleeping pill). Knowing that these effects exist should allow you to take control.

Techniques to help the insomniac

This book provides a framework and context for the use of various techniques. You must do the assessments in Chapter Five before you start using the following techniques. Using the wrong ones may do nothing for your sleep and could make you feel frustrated. There are some tried and tested techniques that in many circumstances will help you sleep. For many years, I have recommended deep breathing exercises (*see pages 120–21*), progressive muscular relaxation exercises (*see pages 122–23*), and others. These will help alleviate anxiety and tension – common factors that contribute to poor sleep.

Occasional use of sleeping pills

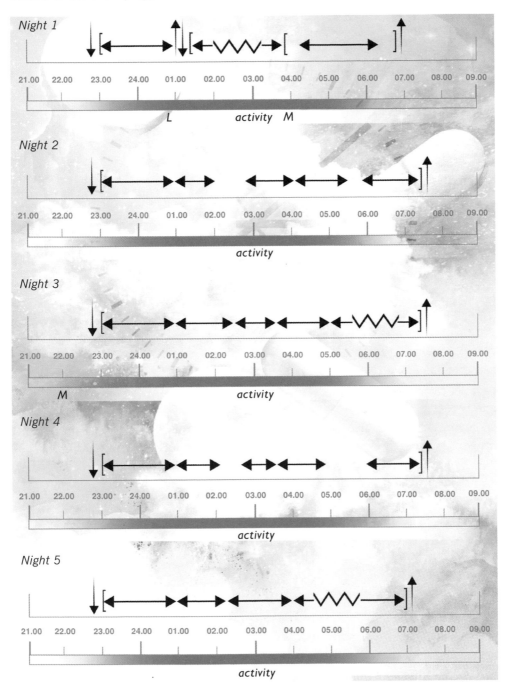

NOW WHAT DO I DO?

Problem	Ruler indications	Action
Alcoholism	Light sleep	Use the diary to get an understanding of your sleep and check the section 'Why can't I fall asleep' (*see page 55*) to ensure that you have not developed other habits or addictions that may be weakening your sleep. Seek further help for your alcohol intake.
Depression	Early-morning waking and/or sleep onset and/or disturbed sleep	Depression is often associated with early-morning waking and fragmented sleep. As with alcoholism, make sure you are not doing anything to weaken your sleep: see 'Why can't I fall asleep?' (*see page 55*). Also, consider the treatment for phase advance (*see page 119*). Seek further help for the depression.
Anxiety	Pre-sleep wakefulness	Anxiety is often associated with muscle tension. Try progressive muscular relaxation (*see pages 122–23*). This technique can be extended by using autogenic training (*see page 124*). See also 'worry-centred insomnia' (*see page 106*). Seek help for further anxiety relief measures.
Social drugs, sleeping pills and medicines	Complex	Learn to understand your sleep and how it may be affected by prescribed, pharmacy, social or abused drugs. See also the section on sleeping pills (*see pages 51–2*).
Worry-centred	Pre-sleep wakefulness and sleep maintenance	Use worry-reduction exercises (*see pages 120–21*), meditation exercises, or thought-blocking techniques such as chanting a mantra. Breathing and relaxation exercises (*see pages 120–22*) will also help.
Tense insomnia	Pre-sleep wakefulness	Try to identify the source of tension: physical (posture, bed, mattress) or mental (reaction to stresses of day). Progressive muscular relaxation or autogenic training (*see pages 122–24*) will help. If anxiety is part of the problem, seek further help for this.

Problem	Ruler indications	Action
Stimulus control insomnia	Pre-sleep wakefulness	If associated with your bed and bedroom, use Bootzin Stimulus Control method (see pages 120–22) to break down the connection.
Insomnia-related	Pre-sleep wakefulness and maintenance	Sleep-centred and worry-centred insomnia often go hand in hand but many chronic insomniacs worry specifically about their sleep. You can use the worry-centred methods listed on the previous page and specific techniques like paradoxical intention (see page 127) but most importantly, challenge your thinking. Do you really cope less well after a bad night? Does everyone see that you haven't slept well? Use the diary in Chapter Five to check.
Phase delay	Pre-sleep	If mild, then simply adjusting wake-up and rise time may be sufficient to increase pressure on sleep. Regularity is important. If more severe, see the section on phase delay (see page 145).
Phase advance	Morning awakenings	If mild, adjusting bedtime, by staying up, may be enough to increase pressure on sleep. Regularity is important. If more severe, see section on phase advance (see page 145).
Snoring	Disturbed sleep	If sleep apnoea is suspected, consult your doctor, especially if daytime sleepiness is severe. See strategies for dealing with snoring and apnoea (see pages 139–40).

Bootzin Stimulus Control

Richard Bootzin, Northwestern University, Chicago, devised this technique more than 40 years ago, to counteract conditioned insomnia.

Problems with falling asleep (young to middle-aged adults)

1. Lie down in your bed to sleep only when feeling sleepy.
2. Use the bed only for sleep (sex is the only exception).
3. If you are unable to sleep in about 20 minutes, get up and ideally leave the bedroom.
4. Return to bed once sleepy and follow instruction 3.
5. Set the alarm to get up at the same time every day.
6. Do not nap during the day.

Problems with falling asleep (adults 60 years and older)

1. Lie down in your bed to sleep only when feeling sleepy.
2. Use the bed only for sleep (sex is the only exception).
3. If you are unable to sleep in about 20 minutes, get up and ideally leave the bedroom.
4. Return to bed once sleepy and follow instruction 3.
5. If you have trouble leaving the bed change your position to a non-sleeping position, e.g. lie on more pillow than usual.

Problems with staying asleep

1. Get up once awake for 10–20 minutes, then follow the falling asleep instructions above.

The purpose of the above instructions is to reduce the association between bed and being awake, to establish an association between bed and falling asleep, and to re-establish the sequence of being sleepy and falling asleep.

Relaxing

The link between muscle tension and sleeplessness has been noted a number of times. Once sleeplessness becomes a problem and problems are faced by increasing tension, then a vicious cycle begins.

Deep breathing

It is easy to become tense through the day. Deep breathing (diaphragmatic breathing) is a well-established relaxation technique. It can be done at almost any time and anywhere.

- If you have never practiced deep breathing, it is best to start on your back.
- Lie down and put one hand on your chest and the other on your abdomen.
- Your legs should either be comfortably outstretched or, if you prefer, bent at the knees with your feet flat on the floor.
- Inhale slowly through the nose.
- Feel the hand on your chest rise.
- When the breath reaches your stomach, push your abdomen upwards, letting your other hand rise slightly higher than the hand on your chest. The abdomen is raised by the diaphragm expanding.
- Hold for one second, then reverse the process. Exhale and allow your muscle to relax and let the air out of your chest and nostrils. Relax your jaw as you exhale.
- As you learn to control your breathing, start concentrating on the breath as you exhale. Appreciate it. Was it smooth, warm, luxurious? How did it feel against your nostrils, your lips? Was it comfortable?
- Sometimes intrusive thoughts will break your concentration on your breathing. Banish them. Don't get angry or frustrated. Think about them as if they were written down on paper. Put the paper in a bottle and throw it into the sea – imagine them floating away.

Do your breathing exercise for 10 minutes twice a day. Try to develop it as a routine. If your body tenses up, do the breathing exercise. Be vigilant to tension. If you become tense, close your eyes and focus on your breathing.

If you have difficulty identifying movement in your stomach, try putting a book on it and force it to go up. Some people find that by doing this, and putting their hands behind their heads, it helps to identify the right muscle to use to execute the movement.

It is best to practice abdominal breathing during the day until you get it right. As you become more proficient, you may feel butterflies in your stomach, or feel as if you are floating. It is worth persevering, as these sensations should become pleasant ones. The more pleasant they become, the more likely you are to go to sleep. If you feel light-headed or dizzy then you may not be breathing fast enough and not enough oxygen is getting into your body. If you are unwell, for whatever reason, it is worth trying the exercise once, for about half an hour and no more. This is to prevent an association developing between the exercise and feelings of frustration and failure.

Variations

Abdominal breathing can be done anywhere, any time, but practicing on your back is usually the easiest way to learn. You could do it in the sitting or standing position, but it is more difficult to feel your abdomen. You can also do the exercise by lying on your stomach with your arms folded in front of your body. Your hands should rest on your biceps. In this position, your chest should not touch the floor. You should feel your abdomen expanding.

On-the-spot deep breathing

You may become aware of your muscles tensing up – this will often happen in your shoulders, back, abdomen or jaw. Deep breathing may help stop the tension developing.

- Inhale slowly, pushing the stomach muscles out.
- Exhale slowly, feeling the stomach muscles collapse.
- As you exhale repeat either a calming or neutral phrase to yourself: for example, 'relax', or, 'quiet' or 'still'. It doesn't matter what the word or phrase is.

Progressive muscular relaxation

Progressive muscular relaxation is useful for problems with going to sleep and problems with returning to sleep after waking up. The muscle groups involved are: hip and legs – feet, calves, thighs, buttocks; torso – lower back, stomach/abdomen, chest; arms – hands, forearms, biceps; head and shoulders – shoulders, neck, throat, head; face – jaws, tongue, lips, nose, cheeks, eyes, brow, scalp.

If you also use the variations (given below), progressive muscular relaxation can take a while to work through – perhaps a month, or even longer. Coupled with other sensible sleep-promoting techniques, it may provide a long-term and enduring solution to your sleep problems.

Variations on progressive muscular relaxation

The technique can be elaborated further by working on both legs or both hands simultaneously. This provides a variation that may prevent the technique from becoming too monotonous or boring. Monotony and boredom are soporific for some but irritating for others.

Yet another variation is to work on diagonal groups of muscles at the same time. This is called differential relaxation. It involves working with two of the major groups of muscles. It could start with tensing the right arm and hand while simultaneously relaxing the left foot and calf, followed by tensing the left foot and calf and relaxing the right hand and arm. This is then followed by tensing the left arm and hand while

Relaxation techniques such as progressive muscular relaxation and autogenic training help to overcome factors that can keep the awake system active, and by doing so, allow sleep to take place.

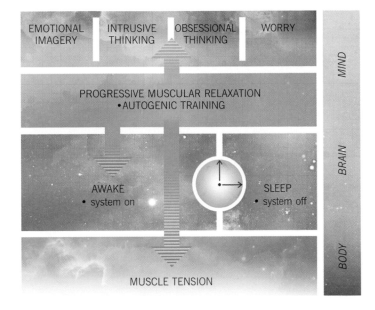

EMOTIONAL IMAGERY | INTRUSIVE THINKING | OBSESSIONAL THINKING | WORRY

PROGRESSIVE MUSCULAR RELAXATION
• AUTOGENIC TRAINING

AWAKE
• system on

SLEEP
• system off

MUSCLE TENSION

MIND

BRAIN

BODY

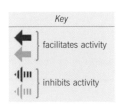

Key

facilitates activity

inhibits activity

simultaneously relaxing the right foot and calf, and finally, relaxing the left arm and hand while tensing the right foot and calf. These routines can also be applied to the other major muscle groups: you can work with any combination.

Autogenic training

Autogenic training uses the same muscle groups as progressive muscular relaxation. It allows you to learn to self-generate feelings of warmth and relaxation. Time must be set aside – at least 20 minutes a day for each main muscle group. Spend a week practicing before trying out this technique in the evening.

Autogenic training routine

Find a quiet spot where you will not be interrupted. The aim is to invoke feelings of warmth and heaviness, and so feel relaxed and ready for sleep. Use a reclining chair, or lie down flat. Wear something loose and comfortable. Take a breath and release it slowly. Another breath and exhale. Another breath and exhale. Your right arm and hand should be lying straight beside you or on the arm of the chair. Concentrate on your muscles and joints, feel their warmth and weight while repeating the phrases (_see page 124_).

AUTOGENIC TRAINING ROUTINE

Once you have followed the preparatory instructions on page 123, you are ready to begin.

- My right hand is feeling heavy.
- My right hand is heavy and warm.
- My right hand is resting.
- My right arm is feeling heavy.
- My right arm is heavy and warm.
- My right arm is resting.

Repeat the above phrases twice. Feel your arm float out on its own, from the shoulders to the elbow to the tips of your fingers.

Now switch to the other side.

- My left hand is feeling heavy.
- My left hand is heavy and warm.
- My left hand is resting.
- My left arm is feeling heavy.
- My left arm is heavy and warm.
- My left arm is resting.

Once you have finished this, and you feel even more relaxed, then stay still for a little while longer. Appreciate the feeling.

After several days of working with arms and hands, you can move on to your legs. Use the same kind of phrases and techniques. You are aiming to elicit feelings of heaviness, lightness or floating.

- My right foot is feeling heavy.
- My right foot is heavy and warm.
- My right foot is resting.
- My right leg is feeling heavy.
- My right leg is heavy and warm.
- My right leg is resting.
- My right thigh is feeling heavy.
- My right thigh is heavy and warm.
- My right thigh is resting.
- My right buttock is feeling heavy.
- My right buttock is heavy and warm.
- My right buttock is resting.

Now switch to the other side.

- My left foot is feeling heavy.
- My left foot is heavy and warm.
- My left foot is resting.
- My left leg is feeling heavy.
- My left leg is heavy and warm.
- My left leg is resting.
- My left thigh is feeling heavy.
- My left thigh is heavy and warm.
- My left thigh is resting.
- My left buttock is feeling heavy.
- My left buttock is heavy and warm.
- My left buttock is resting.

After a few days, you add the next muscle group. Again, the instructions follow the pattern:

- My stomach is feeling heavy.
- My stomach is heavy and warm.
- My stomach is resting.
- My chest is feeling heavy.
- My chest is heavy and warm.
- My chest is resting.
- My lower back is feeling heavy.
- My lower back is heavy and warm.
- My lower back is resting.

Finally, the last group of muscles is added.

- My shoulders are feeling heavy.
- My shoulders are heavy and warm.
- My shoulders are resting.
- My neck and throat are feeling heavy.
- My neck and throat are heavy and warm.
- My neck and throat are resting.
- My head and face are feeling heavy.
- My head and face are heavy and warm.
- My head and face are resting.

Pre-sleep mental exercises and thought blocking

Whether you have a quiet day or a busy day, various thoughts ebb and flow through your mind. These thoughts have to be dealt with, otherwise they may emerge at bedtime. Also, you may fall asleep quickly but wake up later on and the various thoughts of things to do, matters to discuss, appointments to arrange may all flood back. You need to set aside time to deal with these thoughts, so that if they intrude as you try to go to sleep, or if you wake up during the night, you know they have been dealt with.

Before you go to bed, relax and consider what thoughts need to be handled. Think about thoughts that aren't there. Anticipate worrying thoughts. Note them down so that you won't have forgotten them in the morning. If you recall things that you need to do, write them down and remind yourself that you will be able to deal with them after you have slept. And after you have written these notes, stop and think again – are there any others you have forgotten? Write them down. Some people like to visualize their thoughts and then pack them into a box. Close the lid. This exercise should only take 5–10 minutes. Enjoy your uncluttered mind. Use the exercise as part of your bedtime ritual. Teach your body and mind that this is the time for sleep.

Sleep restriction is part of Cognitive-Behavioural Therapy for Insomnia.

WARNING – Legally, you have to look after your alertness. The instructions below deliberately try to reduce the time that you spend awake in bed and make your sleep more efficient. A side effect, particularly initially, may be to cause you to be sleepy. While you may think that is unlikely, you must ensure that you do not do anything that requires you to be fully awake. Driving is an example. It is your responsibility to remain alert. If you are unsure about the instructions, then go to a healthcare professional for guidance.

Instructions

1. Work out the average total time that you sleep in one night. If it is less than 8 hours but greater or equal to 6 hours then proceed to 2. If you sleep less than 6 hours average through the week, consider consulting a healthcare professional.
2. Work out the time that you usually spend in bed. If you spend more time in bed than you sleep then proceed. For example, if you spend 8 hours in bed but sleep only 6 then you should only spend 6 hours in bed. If this is the case then proceed to 3.
3. Plot out the times you fall asleep and wake up for one week (*use the rulers in the Chapter Five diary section*).
4. Circle roughly the times that you go to sleep for the first time and your last awakening (*see example illustration on page 126*).
5. Work out when on average you went to sleep and when you woke up.

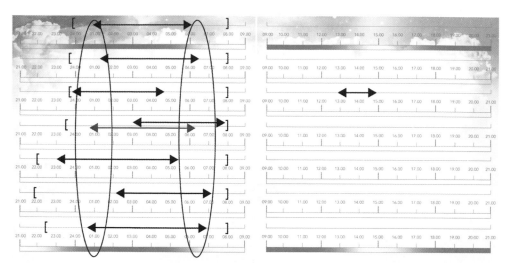

Example of sleep ruler summary.

6. Now go to bed and get up at those times for one week.

7. If you sleep most of the time within the new bed time and awake time then add 15 minutes to the time that you spend in bed. Do this by adding 7.5 minutes at the beginning and end of the night, or go to bed 15 minutes earlier or get up 15 minutes later: whatever suits (or matches your chronotype). If in the next week you are sleeping throughout that time, add another 15 minutes or so and repeat.

8. NO NAPPING!

9. If you are unsure of how to follow these instructions then seek help.

Switching your mind off

People with busy lives often like to use their time in bed to think. That's fine if you can go to sleep when you want, but if you're an insomniac you must use your bed just for sleep. Once you have cleared your mind, try to keep it switched off. A thought for an insomniac is like a drink for an alcoholic – once started, you can't stop. So don't start. Don't over-focus, though, either. If you find you're thinking about not thinking, try to let the thoughts go. Coast; go into neutral.

Final suggestions

You may want to try some additional techniques such as meditation or mentally chanting mantras, but to start off with just try the pre-bed exercises described on the previous page. Don't think deliberately; let your thoughts subside.

Thought blocking

Sometimes your mind will be very active, or you will wake up in the middle of the night with thoughts flooding in. You need to block these thoughts with something neutral that will keep your attention but will not wake you up. One option is simply to repeat a word slowly, such as 'the': the, the, the. It can be any word, something to focus on, but not enough to wake you up. Some people like to visualize a circle with a light attached on the periphery. The light just goes around and around. It's something to occupy the mind.

Paradoxical intention

This is a technique to help you go to sleep. You concentrate on remaining awake and are determined that you will not go to sleep. It helps some people, presumably by blocking out intrusive and alerting thoughts.

Too much caffeine?

If you have worked out that your coffee intake is too high then you must reduce your intake. A reduction of half a cup of coffee per day is managed by most who are addicted, without causing side effects. Use replacements such as hot chocolate or herbal teas. Decaffeinated coffee is not such a good idea, as it is also addictive.

Inappropriate behaviours and beliefs

The questions on sleep-centred insomnia focused on various beliefs about sleep (not coping, poor concentration, feeling unwell) that are often associated with the belief that disturbed sleep causes physical and mental harm. There is little evidence for this. Total sleep deprivation causes transient impairment, but insomniacs actually get their basic biological quota.

Throw out the bedroom clock. It was explained earlier that sleep is normally broken, but most people are not aware of these brief periods of wakefulness. It is quite possible to sleep and wake up without realizing you have been asleep, and to worry about being awake. If you need an alarm clock, turn it round so that you don't look at it.

If you are particularly dissatisfied with the depth of your sleep then read Chapter Seven. Many sleep disorders cause insomnia as well as daytime sleepiness. It is possible that the problem is not insomnia but another condition, such as sleep apnoea.

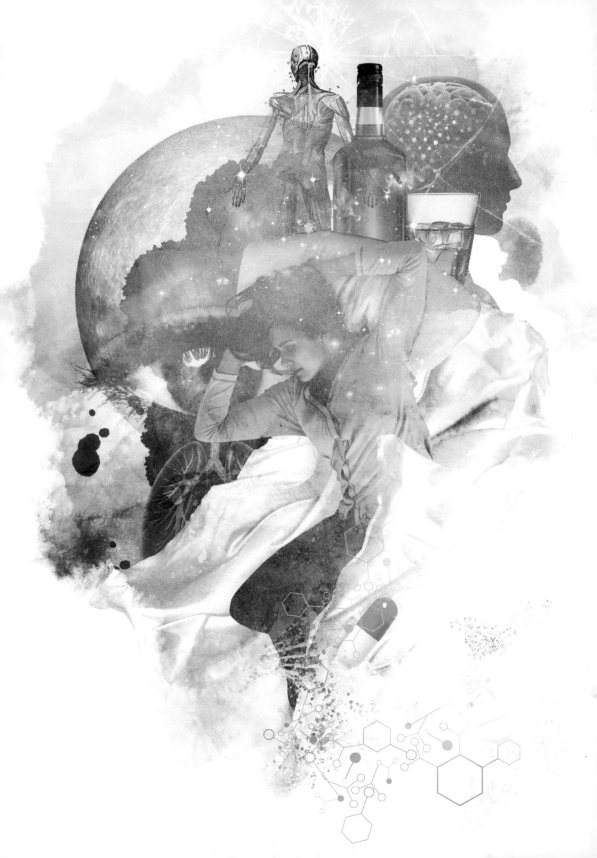

Sleep disorders

. . . .

This book has so far dealt with normal sleep that has been disturbed, either because the individual is somehow mismanaging his or her sleep, or because their role as worker or carer has reduced their ability to cope with disturbed sleep. A good deal of sleeplessness is controllable, but there comes a point when some people may need to seek extra help, because they are suffering from a sleep disorder.

Disordered sleep and sleep disorders

On the basis of three main systems – sleep, awake and clock – this book has described what sleep is, how it works and what goes wrong to create the condition of sleeplessness or insomnia. Other sleep problems can arise too when these systems go wrong with the central sleep, awake and clock systems (sleep disorders), while others are caused when something outside these systems has gone wrong, such as in the case of Parkinson's disease, arthritis, depression, dementia and so on (disordered sleep). Sometimes the categories are not so clearly defined. It is beyond the capacity of this book to deal with all of the alternatives in detail but the currently accepted list can be found in the table overleaf. The main divisions are straightforward: 1) insomnia, 2) sleep-related breathing disorders, 3) hypersomnias – sleepy and not being able to stay awake when you want to 4) parasomnias – undesirable or unwanted behaviours while asleep and 5) sleep-related movement disorders. In this chapter, I will describe the most common disorders.

SLEEP DISORDERS

Type of disorder		Disorder
Insomnia		Chronic Insomnia Disorder
		Short-Term Insomnia
		Other Insomnia
	ISOLATED SYMPTOMS AND NORMAL VARIANTS	Excessive Time in bed
Sleep-related Breathing Disorders	OBSTRUCTIVE SLEEP APNEA DISORDERS	Obstructive Sleep Apnea
		Obstructive Sleep Apnea, Paediatric
	CENTRAL SLEEP APNEA SYNDROMES	Central Sleep Apnea with Cheyne-Stokes Breathing
		Central Apnea Due to a Medical Disorder without Cheyne-Stokes Breathing
		Central Sleep Apnea Due to High-altitude Periodic Breathing
		Central Sleep Apnea Due to a Medication or Substance
		Primary Central Sleep
		Primary Central Sleep Apnea of Infancy
		Primary Central Sleep Apnea of Prematurity
		Treatment-Emergent Central Sleep Apnea
	SLEEP-RELATED HYPOVENTILATION DISORDERS	Obesity Hypoventilation
		Congenital Central Alveolar Hypoventilation Syndrome
		Late-Onset Central Hypoventilation with Hypothalamic Dysfunction
		Idiopathic Central Alveolar Hypoventilation
		Sleep-related Hypoventilation Due to a Medication or Substance
		Sleep-related Hypoventilation Due to a Medical Disorder
Central Disorders of Hypersomnolence		Narcolepsy Type 1
		Narcolepsy Type 2
		Idiopathic Hypersomnia

SLEEP DISORDERS

Type of disorder		Disorder
		Kleine-Levin Syndrome
		Hypersomnia Due to a Medical Disorder
		Hypersomnia Due to a Medication or substance
		Hypersomnia Associated with a Psychiatric Disorder
		Insufficient Sleep Syndrome
	ISOLATED SYMPTOMS AND NORMAL VARIANTS	Long sleeper
Circadian Rhythm Sleep-Wake Disorder		Delayed Sleep-Wake Phase Disorder
		Advanced Sleep-Wake Phase
		Irregular Sleep-Wake Rhythm
		Non-24-Hour Sleep-Wake Rhythm
		Shift Work
		Jet Lag
		Circadian Sleep-Wake Disorder Not Otherwise Specified (NOS)
Parasomnias	NREM-RELATED PARASOMNIAS	Disorders of Arousal (From NREM Sleep)
		Confusional arousals
		Sleepwalking
		Night Terrors
		Sleep-related Eating Disorder
	REM-RELATED PARASOMNIAS	REM Sleep Behaviour
		Recurrent Isolated Sleep
		Nightmare Disorder
	OTHER PARASOMNIAS	Exploding Head Syndrome
		Sleep-related hallucinations
		Sleep
		Parasomnia Due to a Medical Disorder
		Parasomnia unspecified
	ISOLATED SYMPTOMS AND NORMAL VARIANTS	Sleep talking

SLEEP DISORDERS

Type of disorder		Disorder
Sleep-related Movement Disorders		Restless Legs
		Periodic-limb Movement
		Sleep-related Leg Cramps
		Sleep-related Bruxism
		Sleep-related Rhythmic Movement
		Benign Sleep Myoclonus of Infancy
		Propriospinal Myoclonus at Sleep Onset
		Sleep-related Movement Disorder Due to a Medical Disorder
		Sleep-related Movement Disorder Due to a Medication or Substance
		Sleep-related Movement Disorder, unspecified
	ISOLATED SYMPTOMS AND NORMAL VARIANTS	Excessive Fragmentary Myoclonus
		Hypnagogic Foot Tremor and Alternating Leg Muscle Activation
		Sleep Starts (Hypnic Jerks)
Other Sleep Disorders		
Appendix A:		Sleep-related Medical and Neurological Disorders
		Fatal Familial Insomnia
		Sleep-related epilepsy
		Sleep-related headaches
		Sleep-related laryngospasm
		Sleep-related Gastroesophageal reflect
		Sleep-related Myocardial Ischaemia

Sleep disorders centres

There are at least two types of sleep disorders centres: those that concentrate on sleep-related breathing disorders, such as obstructive sleep apnoea (*see page 139*) and those that provide clinical diagnostic services and treatment for all sleep disorders. The latter are usually multidisciplinary and are more likely to have someone with an interest in insomnia. The American Sleep Disorders Association (ASDA) provides an accreditation service for sleep disorders centres and laboratories. The Association ensures that facilities maintain the highest quality of patient care and re-accreditation is required every 5 years. The European Sleep Research Society and the British Sleep Society have also worked on accreditation systems though neither has been as widely adopted as the American one.

What happens when you go to a sleep disorders centre?

Before you go to the centre you will almost certainly receive a diary and questionnaire. This book may have been useful, but the centre will probably want to use its own tests. After a clinical diagnostic interview the decision to have you sleep in the laboratory may be made. Overnight laboratory monitoring involves gluing multiple electrodes (smaller than a five pence coin) onto the scalp to measure brainwaves (on an EEG), eye movement and chin muscle tone. There is no need to be shaved – in fact, bald heads are more difficult as the electrodes tend to skid around when you are trying to apply them! These electrodes provide enough information to identify the main stages of sleep. It is also necessary to measure breathing, as breathing and the level of oxygen in the blood can also disturb sleep. This may involve sensors on the nose (air-flow) and fingers (blood-oxygen levels) and chest-straps (breathing movements). As limb movements can also disturb sleep, further electrodes may also be attached to the legs. This is more or less the standard wiring.

Nowadays, centres will video you during the night as well. This can be helpful in interpreting some of the electrophysiological data and confirming a parasomnia.

This whole procedure is known as nocturnal polysomnography and is the major diagnostic tool in sleep disorders. It is used in the evaluation of periodic limb movement disorder (*see pages 143–44*) and sometimes, depending on the sleep centre, sleep-related breathing disorders. Suspected breathing disorders generally though will start with home monitoring using devices that measure respiratory, heart rate and blood oxygen levels (this is usually only a few electrodes, attachments and chest strap).

Patients often worry about not being able to sleep in the laboratory. The majority do, particularly if their problem is excessive sleepiness. Conditioned insomniacs may also, embarrassingly, sleep well. This should not be a problem as most centres will be aware of both the pitfalls and the benefit of the measurement techniques used.

Many sleep apnoeics (*see page 139*) and narcoleptics (*see pages 137–39*) are very sleepy. The Multiple Sleep Latency Test (MSLT) is used to measure this during the day and simply involves telling the patient to 'Please lie quietly, assume a comfortable position, keep your eyes closed and try to fall asleep' and measuring how long it takes to get to sleep. Narcoleptics may also have a tell-tale sign of REM-sleep onsets. If the issue is remaining awake while working then a different test is used: The Multiple Wake Test. This is the same as the MSLT except the instructions are to remain awake for as long as possible (extraordinary measures like sleeping on one's face are not allowed!).

Insomnia

In the introduction I described the ways insomnia was formally redefined over the years. The essentials are always the same, not being able to sleep when you want to even though it is reasonable that you should be able to sleep and that inability is causing distress and functional problems. The changes in definition reflect the difficulty science is having with categorizing the problem. The changes are summarized in the diagram opposite.

Psychophysiological insomnia

Psychophysiological insomnia is also known as learned insomnia or conditioned insomnia. As with many chronic insomnia it is thought to arise in susceptible individuals after some precipitating event. The event may be minor – perhaps not being able to adjust quickly after jet lag, or after a bereavement, or even after a change of job. There is usually one point in time that the patient can identify when their sleep deteriorated. There is an obvious precipitating factor. There are usually other factors associated with chronic insomnia which tend to perpetuate the situation. These may arise as a result of trying to cope with the insomnia, or they may always have been present. Many of the factors harmful to good sleep were identified in Chapters Three and Four. Napping is not necessarily the wrong thing to do in this situation, though chronic insomniacs often cannot take naps: whatever keeps them awake during the night also keeps them awake during the day.

Conditioned insomniacs often react to stress by increasing muscle tension, which makes it difficult to fall asleep. On top of this, they also become very focused on their sleep. This creates a nasty cycle of events: they try to sleep, fail, become tense, fail

Insomnia: redefined

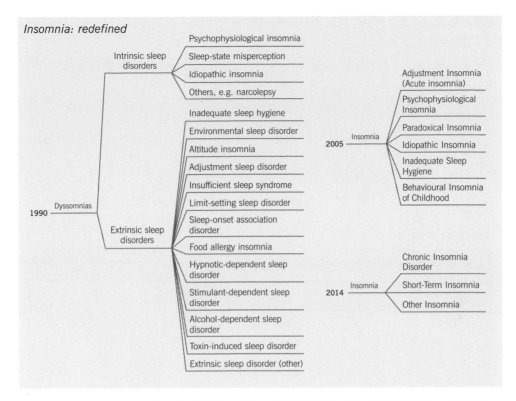

Sleep medicine continues to refine the definition of sleep. 2014 is simpler than 1990! 1990 is particularly helpful as it identifies different possible causes. The latest definitions lump a lot of 'insomnias' together: the reason given is that they were difficult to identify and did not have much effect on treatment. I only partly agree so I still use some of the types that were recognized in earlier versions.

again, become tenser and have considerable difficulties ever getting to sleep (*see diagram on page 136*). A learned association between failing to sleep and the bedroom exacerbates their difficulties. Chapter Six covered some of the techniques that can be used to deal with conditioned insomnia, such as the Bootzin Stimulus Control (*see page 120*) and the breathing and relaxation exercises. The techniques will work, but if insomnia has become ingrained, and possibly complicated with sleeping-pill dependence, then the help of an expert therapist should be considered.

Paradoxical insomnia (Sleep-state misperception)

This diagnosis occurs when a patient claims not to have slept at all, yet polysomnography carried out at a sleep centre indicates that they did. This is a rare situation. Peter Hauri (Mayo Clinic) reports one patient who dreamed that he was awake trying to sleep!

Conditioned insomniacs experience a perpetual cycle of trying to sleep, failing, becoming tense and agitated, their minds filling with negative thoughts, then falling asleep, only to awaken to become tense and agitated again, and so on.

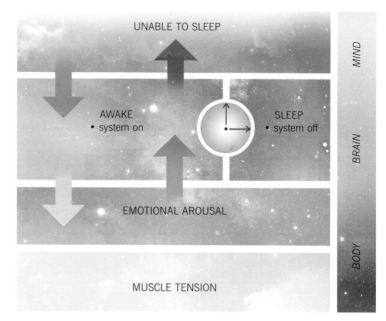

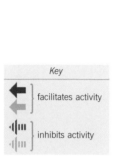

Key

facilitates activity

inhibits activity

Idiopathic insomnia

This insomnia is also known as childhood onset insomnia. It is a lifelong inability to get adequate sleep and presumably reflects an underactive sleep system or an overactive awake system. This insomnia is unremitting, but the mental state of the sufferer generally remains good. There are no events that trigger this: as far as the patient recalls, he or she has tended to be alert most of the time. Polysomnography shows very poorly formed EEG sleep that is clearly unusual. Treatment involves two simultaneous strategies: first, all the methods described in previous chapters have to be employed to increase the possibility of sleep; and secondly, low-dose sedating antidepressants are given (sleeping pills only work occasionally). The low-dose antidepressant is well below the dose required to act as an antidepressant, but these compounds have multiple pharmacological actions, some of which appear to be both beneficial and long-lasting.

Excessive sleep and daytime sleepiness

Some people have problems controlling their sleep. Unfortunately, in many societies, past and present, they have been labelled as lazy. The National Commission on Sleep Disorders Research reported in 1993 that inappropriate sleepiness during the day cost the US over $15 billion in direct expenses and nearly $70 billion dollars in lost productivity. Telling someone that he or she is lazy is not enough.

Narcolepsy

The rulers on page 138 show an individual who has disturbed sleep and naps frequently during the day. These naps are extremely difficult to resist and are occasionally irresistible. The pattern of dreaming is also unusual, as dreams are reported at the beginning of sleep.

Narcolepsy

Narcolepsy is generally inherited – close relatives are 60 times more likely to have narcolepsy and genetic markers have been identified. It usually develops in late adolescence or early adulthood. The symptoms often emerge slowly. Unfortunately, an increased incidence of narcolepsy was also observed after the H1N1 flu vaccination (and possibly infection).

It is an underactive-wake-system abnormality over which the narcoleptics have no control. It is thought that it is an autoimmune or immune response usually triggered by an infection targeting those cells in genetically predisposed individuals.

The main symptoms are daytime sleepiness and sudden bouts of muscle weakness, possibly paralysis (often experienced either immediately after an intense emotion, whether it be just laughing or just before falling asleep). Frightening hallucinations can occur at sleep onset, although sometimes it is more of a confusion between knowing whether you are awake and doing something, or dreaming about doing something. Some sufferers can go into automatic mode for many minutes and then not recall that they are awake. An irony for narcoleptics is that they can often also suffer from sleep-lessness during the night.

When given the Multiple Sleep Latency Test (MSLT) narcoleptics fall asleep very quickly. An unusual feature of their sleep is that it often begins with REM sleep. This occurs at night as well as on some of the MSLT tests. REM occurring at sleep onset and the muscle paralysis point to something going wrong with the REM control system of the sleep system (see pages 34–5).

Narcolepsy does not appear to be common but estimates of numbers in the US range from 100,000–600,000. It is often left undiagnosed. Narcoleptics are often labelled as lazy and many have problems holding onto their jobs. Those suffering from mild narcolepsy do not like to admit that sometimes they are not sure whether they are

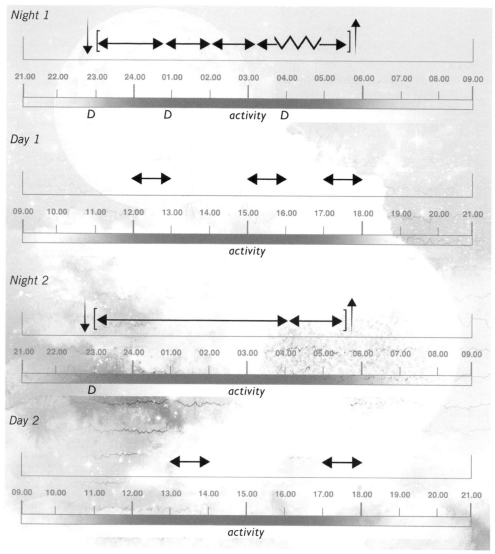

Narcolepsy

awake or dreaming. For adolescents and youngsters this can be particularly frightening. Narcolepsy can be treated to a great extent using stimulants such as amphetamines and modafinil and antidepressants (again, antidepressants are not being used to control depression) but to control the muscle paralysis. Taking scheduled naps during the day also reduces the need to sleep and so lessens the number of episodes of uncontrolled sleep. Loss of muscle control can be associated with strong emotions, such as deep joy or anger. This onset of muscle weakness prepares the narcoleptic for a sleep episode, so he or she can try to keep it under control.

Snoring and sleep apnoea

Sleep apnoea is diagnosed when someone stops breathing during sleep. The partner will almost certainly be aware of the snoring (sometimes the noise-level of snoring can approach industrial levels of noise pollution!) and will probably have noticed periods when the sleeper has stopped breathing. It is not clear yet whether snoring or sleep apnoea and the resulting lowering of blood-oxygen levels and/or the disrupted sleep are associated with grave medical consequences (studies to disambiguate this are still being conducted). However, sleep apnoea (and possibly snoring) are certainly associated with a greatly increased incidence of highway accidents. The danger from sleep apnoea is undeniable – unexpected and involuntary sleep. Highway driving is not kind to the sleepy. Shiftworkers, including nurses and doctors and sleep apneics are all involved in accidents, sometimes fatal, more often than those whose sleep is not impaired.

In obstructive sleep apnoea, a blockage stops breathing. As the respiratory system detects lowered oxygen levels it increases the muscular effort involved in breathing. As levels drop, increased attempts are made to breathe and the awake system is drawn in to aid the situation. Sleep begins to lighten. In a major episode, wakefulness may result, but it may be of such a short duration that the person is unaware that he or she has been awake. In more minor episodes, the EEG may not show wakefulness, but it does usually show some activity. These minor disruptions are sufficient to impair sleep so that the person is sleepy the next day.

HOW SLEEP APNOEA CAUSES SLEEPINESS
Breathing stops, causing increased arousal and a move towards wakefulness.

↓

The increased arousal causes breathing to restart without conscious awareness returning. However, sleep has been impaired, resulting in increased sleepiness.

Snoring in adults and children

Snoring is often viewed as amusing, but it can lead to marital or partnership discord. Here are some tips on how to reduce snoring (and possibly sleep apnoea):

- Don't drink alcohol within 5 hours of going to bed.
- Avoid taking sleeping pills and tranquilizers.
- Stop smoking.
- If necessary, lose weight.
- Try sleeping on your side rather than your back.
- Improve nasal breathing.
- Raise the head of the bed.
- An improvement in breathing can be produced by trying a different position during sleep as well as by using a nasal decongestant.
- Use nasal decongestants which do not contain ephedrine or pseudoephedrine (both of these will keep you awake).
- If you are suffering from hayfever, take non-sedating antihistamines to clear the airways.
- Nasal dilators or other devices are sometimes useful as well.

Snoring in children should be taken seriously, particularly if they are sleepy during the day (or are hyperactive), aggressive and have learning difficulties. Research has found that children with recurring tonsillitis and this pattern of behaviour benefit from the surgical removal of their tonsils. Both daytime and night-time behaviour resolve and growth spurt may also occur.

Breathing movements might not stop with mild obstructive sleep apnoea. In more severe cases patients' breathing may stop, to the extent that their partners are alarmed and wake them up to restart their breathing. Breathing often restarts with loud snores, mumbling noises and grunting. Body movements also usually occur and sufferers are often described as restless sleepers. Going to the lavatory to urinate also occurs more often as symptoms progress.

When sleep apnoeic patients wake up, they generally feel unrefreshed and are possibly disoriented, uncoordinated and groggy. Morning headaches, which clear up one to two hours after waking up, are a common feature. Stories of laziness, lost jobs and broken marriages abound. Naps are generally not refreshing, in contrast to narcoleptics, who find naps refreshing.

Epworth Sleepiness Scale

Dr Murray Johns of Melbourne, Australia, designed and validated the Epworth Sleepiness Scale (ESS). It asks a patient to rate the chance of dozing during various daytime activities. Fill in the chart below and then answer the questions in the chart on page 142.

After completing the table, review how many questions have been answered yes. If the majority are yes then you may well be suffering from sleep apnoea. If a few are yes, but particularly if you are a middle-aged male, with a collar size greater than 42 cm (17 in), who is overweight, snores and is sleepy during the day (Epworth score 10 or greater), then you are likely to be suffering from sleep apnoea.

Therapy for apnoea

Therapies can be conservative: weight reduction, stopping smoking, avoiding alcohol and sleeping pills – in fact, many of the suggestions listed in the snoring section of this chapter (*see page 139*) but it must be taken seriously. Go to your GP to get a referral to a sleep centre! Sometimes apnoeas are dependent on sleeping position and adjusting

Epworth Sleepiness Scale

In contrast to just feeling tired, how likely are you to doze off or fall asleep in the following situations? (Even if you have not done some of these things recently, try to work out how they would affect you.) Use the following scale to choose the most appropriate number for each situation:

0 = would never doze   1 = slight chance of dozing   2 = moderate chance of dozing
3 = high chance of dozing

Situation	Chance of Dozing
1. Sitting reading	
2. Watching TV	
3. Sitting inactive in a public place (such as the theatre)	
4. As a car passenger for an hour without a break	
5. Lying down to rest in the afternoon	
6. Sitting talking to someone	
7. Sitting quietly after lunch without alcohol	
8. In a car, while stopping for a few minutes in traffic	
Total Score	

0–8: normal sleep function • 8–10: mild sleepiness • 11–15: moderate sleepiness
16–20: severe sleepiness • 21–24: excessive sleepiness

Sleep apnoea assessment

Questions	Yes	No
Physical condition		
Are you overweight?		
Do you have high blood pressure?		
Do you have trouble breathing through your nose?		
Do you often have a drink of alcohol before going to bed?		
If you are a man, is your collar size 42 cm (17 in) or larger?		
During the night		
Do you snore loudly each night?		
Have you been told that you stop breathing for 10 seconds or more when you are asleep?		
Are you a restless sleeper?		
Do you have to get up several times to urinate?		
Waking up		
Do you wake up in the morning tired and 'foggy', not ready to face the day?		
Do you have headaches in the morning?		
Are you very sleepy during the day?		
During the day		
Do you have difficulty concentrating and completing tasks?		
Do you carry out routine tasks in a daze?		
Have you ever arrived home in your car but could not remember the trip from work?		
Emotional life		
Are you having serious relationship problems at home, with friends and relatives or at work?		
Are you afraid that you may be out of touch with the real world, unable to think clearly, losing your memory or emotionally ill?		
Are you irritable and angry, especially first thing in the morning?		

the sleep position may benefit some sufferers. There are no widely accepted pharmacological preparations.

Nasal-CPAP (continuous positive airway pressure) is the most common treatment. This involves devices that blow air into the airways at a pressure sufficient to keep the airways open. These devices have been called pneumatic splints. The impact for the patient is almost immediate and usually overnight – they will know when they've been treated successfully. Nasal-CPAP is well tolerated, particularly if the mask is well fitted and you have a good nurse/technician who does the fitting, although some patients or their partners may not find it acceptable. Various surgical and dental treatments do exist, but there is still some doubt as to the efficacy of these treatments. Mandibular advancement devices may work and can be fitted by dentists.

Restless-legs syndrome

Someone suffering from restless-legs syndrome (RLS aka Wilis-Ekbom disease) feels as if they need to move their legs. There is often an uncomfortable creeping and crawling or pins and needles sensation deep within the legs or running up and down the legs. This sensation occurs while awake, usually in the evening at bedtime, or during sleep. The movement required to alleviate this feeling may have to be quite vigorous.

Individuals suffering from restless-legs syndrome almost invariably suffer from periodic limb movement (see below) but not vice versa. Addiction to caffeine, uraemia and anaemia should be considered as causes of leg discomfort.

Periodic limb movement disorder

Periodic limb movement disorder (PLMD) usually affects the legs. It is different to the sleep starts that occur at the onset of drowsiness prior to sleep. The toe extends and the ankle (and possibly, knees and hips) flex a little. The movements occur every 15–40 seconds and can be grouped into runs of half a minute to an hour. Individuals may not be aware that these movements are taking place and can report unrefreshing sleep or insomnia, or daytime sleepiness. Bed partners may report kicking. The movements can be sufficient to prevent sleep reaching the deeper stages. If the EEG is examined, it can be seen that conscious awareness will not result from this type of disruption even though sleep itself is disturbed.

Patients with sleep apnoea may move their limbs periodically, but these movements often disappear when the sleep apnoea is treated. Also, patients with epilepsy may have periodic limb movements, but again these are different to those found in periodic limb-movement disorder.

Periodic limb movements and restless legs often occur together and apart from being found in sleep apnoea are also often found in narcolepsy. It is not clear why this should be. The current speculation is that these disorders involve damage to roughly the same areas of the brain.

Patients with RLS and PLMD may experience insomnia, fatigue and daytime sleepiness. The cause of the daytime sleepiness is similar to that found in sleep apnoea, meaning that the limb movements are sufficient to disrupt sleep without necessarily causing conscious waking. The sufferer is more likely to complain of insomnia if they do become conscious during the limb movements.

Periodic limb movement has been associated with renal disorders and patients on dialysis may suffer more than most. There are also associations with iron-deficiency anaemia, muscle disorders, peripheral neuron disorders, diabetes, rheumatoid arthritis, chronic-fatigue syndrome, and fibromyalgia. Pregnancy often makes the disorder worse. Sleep polysomnography is most useful in confirming the diagnosis of RLS or PLMD and whether it is associated with any other sleep disorders.

Treatments currently include a number of different pharmacological approaches. Clonazepam or other benzodiazepines may be prescribed, or levodopa/carbidopa or bromocriptine, or various opioids (codeine, methadone, oxycodone, propoxyphene) may be tried before the right drug is found. Iron supplements, where a deficiency is noted, may be useful in elderly patients.

Circadian disorders

Sleeping difficulties that are related to problems with the biological clock are termed circadian disorders. The symptoms and problems are similar to those described in the sections on jet lag and shiftwork, but they do not disappear by themselves. If serious enough, both jet lag and shiftwork may be diagnosed as disorders. The sufferer has a perpetual problem without treatment. These disorders often present themselves as insomnia or excessive daytime sleepiness. Without a diary or actigraph it may not be immediately obvious that a circadian disorder is present. Prescription of sleeping pills is not helpful as it is often associated with increasing usage. Self-medication with alcohol and stimulants such as tobacco is common.

Phase delay: phase advance

Phase delay (also known as delayed-sleep-phase syndrome) is a problem that may be caused by the biological clock not being reset in the mornings. It causes progressively later and later bedtimes until social constraints, such as going to school or going to work, force the sleeper to get up. In the morning the sufferer is very drowsy because he or she is partially sleep-deprived and because the circadian rhythm of alertness is still set for night-time sleep. As the day progresses they feel more and more alert, and this alertness is maintained in the evenings. Sufferers consistently complain of not being able to get to sleep at desirable bedtimes and they often do not go to bed until after midnight, sometimes 02:00–03:00.

Absenteeism is a common result. Many individuals end up doing night work as they cannot keep daytime jobs. The pattern of delayed sleep often develops early in life but becomes evident either at school or work. Individuals invariably sleep well on holiday when there is no definite time to get up. This is a treatable disorder, but ideally, it should be managed by a sleep disorders centre. Chronotherapy, bright light and medications provide a wide variety of treatment possibilities.

Phase advance, which causes earlier and earlier bedtimes and getting up times, is also a clock disorder, often seen in the elderly. It is more likely to affect your social life than your work. Again, this is treatable by a sleep disorders centre.

Non-24-hour sleep-awake syndrome and irregular sleep-awake pattern

Two other clock disorders have been described: non-24-hour sleep-awake syndrome, and irregular sleep-awake pattern. In the former, sleep is delayed in a manner similar to phase-delay syndrome, but the 1–2 hour delays continue and are unremitting. The cycle length appears to be between 25 and 27 hours, and social and environmental cues fail to synchronize the sleep-awake pattern. Sleeping pills and stimulants rarely work. Many patients suffering from this syndrome give up trying to synchronize their sleep with socially acceptable times. Patients whose blindness has been caused by the complete destruction of the retina or severance of their optic nerves may suffer from this disorder as light-dark information is not being transmitted to the biological clock. Irregular sleep-awake pattern has no discernible cyclicity: neither 24-hour nor 90-minute cycles are evident. This can occur in elderly, possibly demented, and institutionalized patients.

Parasomnias

Parasomnias are usually undesirable or unusual behaviours associated with sleep. They occur exclusively within the sleep state and most are associated with either slow-wave sleep (deep sleep) or REM sleep. In terms of the sleep, awake and clock systems, the sleep system is working but its orchestration and control of other brain events is incomplete. The parasomnias are subdivided into arousal disorders (such as sleepwalking), parasomnias associated with REM sleep and other parasomnias.

Arousal disorders

Arousal usually refers to physiological or cortical (brain) activation. Originally, these disorders comprized sleepwalking (somnambulism), night terrors, nocturnal enuresis and nightmare. Since then nocturnal enuresis and nightmare have been redefined. Sleepwalking and night terrors occur in slow-wave sleep, whereas nightmares arise in REM sleep. Nocturnal enuresis can occur at any stage of sleep.

These disorders involve behaviours that are not fully controlled by conscious awareness. In fact, conscious awareness may not return until after the behaviours have stopped. There is invariably confusion and little response to the environment or people. It is very difficult to wake the sleeper and more often than not, he or she does not recall what was happening.

Confusional arousals

Other names for confusional arousals are sleep drunkenness or excessive sleep inertia. They typically occur out of slow-wave sleep but are much less dramatic than sleepwalking or night terrors. The person is often disoriented and will talk and think very slowly. There may be inappropriate behaviour and inappropriate use of objects. Children may cry. These arousals are similar to the other disorders of arousal in that they occur mainly in children, decline with adolescence and usually disappear in adulthood. Although disconcerting, they are harmless.

Sleepwalking

Sleepwalking usually begins abruptly. The sleeper sits up in bed with a relatively blank expression on his or her face. When the sleeper gets up, he or she may adjust the bed and pillow and walk around the room. Some of the movements are clumsy and purposeless. However, many complex acts have been described, such as playing a musical instrument, eating and drinking – even trying to phone someone. Episodes usually last about 10 minutes. Talking coherently is rare. Generally the person is very unresponsive, probably because they are still in slow-wave sleep, or just out of slow-wave sleep. This stage is very deep and much of the brain is involved in this activity that appears not to be involved in any information processing. Waking is difficult but not dangerous, although sleepwalkers may resist attempts to wake up!

Despite the lack of response, sleepers do negotiate furniture relatively easily. Eating while sleepwalking seems to occur quite often and in fact is now known as a separate sleep disorder: sleep-related eating disorder. One case involved a woman who used to sleepwalk to the fridge and consume substantial amounts of food. Interestingly, she was also phobic to snakes and treatment was eventually successful when a model snake was put in front of the fridge. This was sufficient to induce a change of mind and she went back to bed! Also, it is arguable that sleep-related sexual behaviour is an appetitive disorder. The prevalence of this behaviour is not clear – it may be quite high, given the prevalence of dream-enactment behaviour.

Most reported sleepwalking occurs between the age of 5 and adolescence, peaking around age 12. Sleepwalking does not usually go on beyond 12 years. Between 15 and 30 per cent of children sleepwalk and 3 per cent are frequent sleepwalkers. Both sexes are represented. In adults, there are suspicions that the occurrence of sleepwalk-ing is greater than the 1 per cent that is reported in most textbooks, but data is lacking. There are virtually no reports of sleepwalking in pregnant women. There is a strong inheritance factor, with 80 per cent of sleepwalkers having relatives who sleepwalk as well. Sleeptalking also occurs more often in sleepwalkers.

Stress, various medications and alcohol can trigger bouts of sleepwalking. It is not a psychiatric disorder: it just reflects how the brain is organized and how various parts shut down (or not) during sleep. Children who sleepwalk can be triggered into walking by standing them up when they are deeply asleep.

Sleepwalking must be diagnosed accurately as other neurological disorders can cause similar activity. The general advice is to protect sleepwalkers because they can injure themselves. There are various medicines for the physician to try and growing evidence that the activating SSRI class of antidepressants may be useful. Finally, don't panic. It is very difficult to wake up someone who is sleepwalking, but it does them no harm if you must. Just don't expect to be thanked.

Night (sleep) terrors

Night terrors are an abrupt waking out of slow-wave sleep (deep sleep), similar to sleepwalking, but are associated with a loud piercing scream or some other loud noise. Arguably, a night terror can be more frightening for the observer than the person experiencing it, as the sleeper rarely recalls the event. The scream can be associated with various repetitive movements: arms may flail about, there can be intense sweating, hair can stand up, the pupils may be dilated and breathing may be rapid and shallow. The movements in a night terror might also involve the sleeper jumping out of bed, running out of the bedroom and being injured in the process.

The whole episode can last about 15 minutes without the person ever really waking up. Mixtures of behaviour can occur. The sleeper may be talking about what's happening one second and be fast asleep the next. Sufferers rarely recall the event the next day. For youngsters aged between 5 and 7, these episodes can occur roughly once a week. In younger children it may be as often as once a night. Two-thirds of children will have stopped by adolescence. Night terrors are unusual in adults and there is a strong inheritance factor: 96 per cent of sufferers have a family history.

The factors that trigger night terrors are similar to sleepwalking, namely stress, psychoactive compounds and, in adults, alcohol. In children, night terrors do not imply that there is an underlying psychiatric or neurological problem, but simply reflect a maturing brain. In adults, however, since night terrors are rare, precipitating factors as well as underlying problems should be evaluated. As individuals suffering from night terrors seem fully in fight or flight mode, it is important to ensure that they don't injure themselves. There is no effective and safe treatment available.

There is another unusual disorder that may be linked to night terrors: unexplained nocturnal death syndrome. It is not clear whether this syndrome, which is most often found in South-east Asian refugees, arises in slow-wave sleep or REM sleep. Night terrors are associated with a massive increase in heart rate and it has been postulated that this might trigger precipitous death in these individuals. Equally, in REM sleep, heart rate and respiration are less rigorously controlled than during wakefulness and other stages of sleep.

Parasomnias usually related to REM sleep

These behaviours are associated particularly with REM sleep. REM is usually a time of muscle paralysis (apart from breathing), a time when autonomic functions (breathing, heart rate, sweating and other temperature regulation mechanisms) are less well regulated and when the sexual apparatus is unrestrained. If awoken during REM, sleep the individual usually reports bizarre stories with varying amounts of visual imagery. Most disorders involve a REM component failure.

Nightmares

Nightmares usually consist of long and complicated dreams that become more and more frightening. The awakening is associated with immediate recall of the dream and the person can be quite lucid about the experience – this contrasts strongly with night terrors.

Between 10–50 per cent of children suffer from nightmares between the ages of 3 and 6. The incidence grows with age and then usually declines without active intervention, other than providing comfort and support. Dream content is variable and the anxiety that is provoked is purely subjective.

Nightmares occur in both girls and boys, but two to four times more women are affected in adulthood. Approximately 50 per cent of adults admit to having an occasional nightmare. One per cent of the population may have a nightmare every week.

Nightmares are frequently observed in those suffering from post-traumatic stress disorder (PTSD). This disorder can arise after any traumatic event, both civilian and military, although military casualties have been studied most. Many Second World War veterans still suffer from anxiety dreams. In this older group, there may also be failures in breathing. The episodes of sleep apnoea may cause an increase in autonomic and then emotional arousal that intrudes into the REM state. The emotional arousal then drives the content of the dream. Treatment of nightmares varies. Medical practitioners may try prescribing drugs that reduce REM sleep with varying success. In PTSD, cognitive and behavioural methods that help the individual in controlling the anxiety associated with the dream imagery can be quite successful.

Sleep paralysis

The American neurologist Weir Mitchell reported two cases of sleep paralysis in 1876. As the name suggests, it involves waking up and not being able to move. It arises because of a mistiming between the systems that control the muscle paralysis of REM sleep and those that control wakefulness (*see page* 35). You wake up before you can move – it can be very frightening. It occurs rarely in normal individuals (once in a lifetime in 40–50 per cent of the population), can run in families, is often associated with narcolepsy and may occasionally be seen in obstructive sleep apnoea.

The person afflicted can move the eyes and most of the muscles involved in breathing are unaffected – but some might be and this can give rise to feelings of suffocation. Most episodes only run for 1–2 minutes. Once experienced, most people realize if it happens again that sleep paralysis is not life-threatening. It can be more disturbing if it lasts longer, as the individual tends to drift in and out of dreams as well. In Victorian times sleep paralysis was regarded as so frightening by some that they asked for their wrists to be cut when they died, to avoid being buried alive. Sleep paralysis is similar to the medical condition cataplexy and pharmacological treatments are similar.

REM behaviour disorder

REM behaviour disorder is almost the opposite of sleep paralysis, in that the mechanism controlling muscle paralysis does not work. Any movement in dreams is then acted out. The condition appears to occur in men more than women. It has only been fully described in recent years.

Episodes are rare to start with, but the frequency appears to increase over time. Patients may complain about the disorder to their doctor, but they are more likely to complain about daytime sleepiness first. Their partner may well be aware of their difficulties. The movements can be very dramatic, involving leaping and jumping out of bed. Some patients have been reported to have themselves tied down to their beds or have themselves tied into sleeping bags so that they do not injure themselves or anyone else.

REM behaviour disorder can be controlled using a particular benzodiazepine called clonazepam. The reason for its peculiar efficacy is unknown.

Other parasomnias

Nocturnal enuresis

Enuresis (from the Greek word for 'to urinate') is involuntary urination. Nocturnal enuresis just means wetting the bed at an age when this is not expected. Enuresis is subdivided into two types: secondary enuresis describes the onset of night-time wetting three or more months after night-time dryness has been established, whereas primary enuresis refers to someone who has never had a dry night. The age at which night-time dryness emerges depends on a number of factors: sex, pattern of wetting and cultural background.

Toilet training usually follows a pattern of daytime control of urination, followed by daytime bowel control, followed by night-time bowel control and finally night-time bladder control. Control is achieved by the majority of children between 3 and 5 years old, but 15 per cent of 5-year-olds still wet the bed. Generally, older children suffer from primary enuresis, because the development of control has never completed. However, secondary enuresis, once established, may take 1–2 years to abate. Young adults may also develop secondary enuresis. The incidence of enuresis in military populations is high: 20 per cent.

Nocturnal enuresis should be regarded as a benign, although inconvenient, event. As always, some investigation is appropriate as it may be a symptom of a neurological disorder, but it should not be considered as a psychiatric disorder. It may be amenable to behavioural treatments, using conditioning devices that wake the sufferer when the urine triggers a sensor. Bladder training involves increasing fluids during the day so as to stretch the bladder and reducing intake prior to sleep. There are also training programs to increase awareness of the sphincter muscles that control urination. The cause of the problem is still being investigated, but one of the strong possibilities is that not enough anti-diuretic hormone is secreted during the night. This hormone normally reduces urine production, so more is produced than the bladder can control.

Sleep bruxism

Bruxism, or tooth-grinding, may start when teeth erupt, continue into adolescence and can even occur in the elderly who have artificial teeth as well as the completely toothless. It occurs most in light sleep (stage 2) and can be accompanied by slow eye movements. It is often associated with stress. There are numerous hypotheses concerning the mechanisms involved and equally numerous treatments. Night-guards at least protect the teeth.

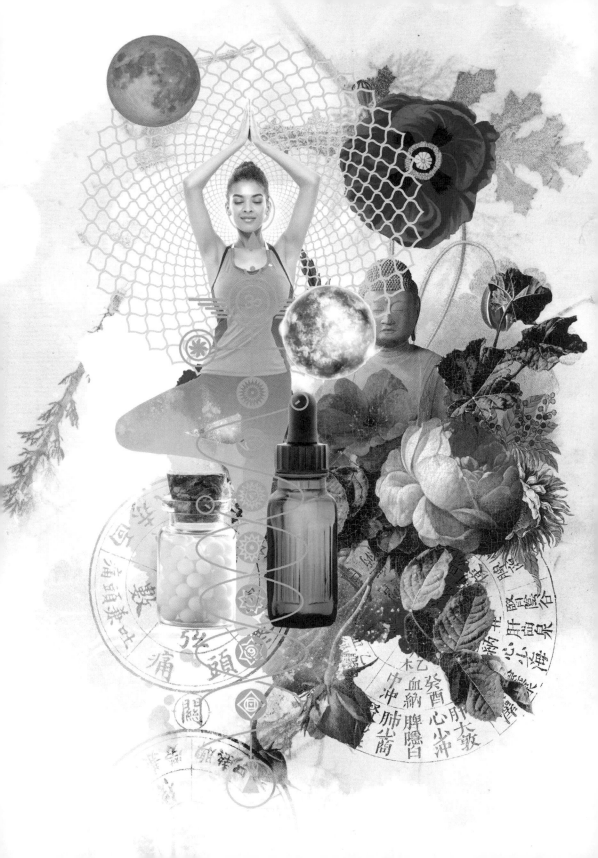

CHAPTER EIGHT

Using complementary therapies

. . . .

This chapter outlines many of the complementary forms of healing and medicine that are said to affect sleep, or claim to treat insomnia or other sleep disorders. The danger in gathering together all these techniques in one chapter is that equal weight is apparently given to each one, but this is not intended. Chinese medicine and yoga, for example, have many thousands of years of tradition and practice behind them, whereas biorhythms, biofeedback and hypnotherapy are relatively new to the healing professions.

All the complementary and alternative techniques have methodological problems in the studies that have been conducted so I cannot definitively say one way or another which to try. It's best to read the early chapters to understand how sleep is controlled and then read about the alternatives available. If the hypothetical mechanisms for those practices or treatments match you, then try them out. Ideally, consult a practitioner if you can afford one and definitely consult a herbalist if you are thinking of trying any of the herbs (none of which actually had solid evidence in the scientific reviews) and see how you get on. Remember the placebo effect (and I'm not saying any of these therapies rely on placebo effects) is real and adopting a practice may doubly benefit you – placebo plus any benefits of the practice. Remember to use the diary as nearly all the treatments take time to take effect. I should also mention physical activity here – that's all I'm going to say, you do need to keep active!

Is it OK to use non-conventional techniques?

The answer is to consult with your doctor: there is no general advice. Your GP should be able to advise you, assuming he or she knows the treatment. Most doctors take the view that alternative treatments are worth trying, provided they are not likely to do you any harm and do not prevent you from using a conventional therapy that works.

Insomnia

Adult sleep is a learned behaviour and is an amalgamation of three controlling brain systems: sleep, awake and clock. For industrialized societies, the learning consists of identifying night-time (darkness) and the biological clock time so that the awake system runs down and the sleep system fires up. Whether someone sleeps on a particular night depends on his or her physical status (feeling well, ill or in pain), mental status (worrying, depressed or anxious), environment (noisy family and so on) and how well learned is the association of darkness with sleep

The chart on the following pages lists a variety of techniques claimed to have beneficial effects on sleep, making one wonder whether everything promotes sleep. This is quite likely. Many disturbances and disorders disrupt sleep, so many of these remedies may affect sleep by minimizing the disruption, rather than by any direct effect on sleep. Also, the definition of insomnia is still in a process of refinement. But for the sufferer, none of this matters – whether it works is far more important than why it works. The treatments featured in the chart can be grouped into the following categories.

Ingestions (herbs, minerals and hormones)

Eating or drinking something for a sleep problem has been a 'cure' from time immemorial. The reason for taking a particular herb, mineral or hormone varies depending on which system of herbalism is used. Minerals that can be obtained from drug stores and health-food shops are also listed, including melatonin. Taking drugs, minerals, herbs and the like is rather like pouring gasoline over a car and hoping that some of it gets into the engine, so you should be wary of other effects than the one that is desired.

Thought management and anxiety relief

Worrying or arousing thoughts prevent sleep, so any method that absorbs your attention may allow sleep to cut in. Some methods were introduced earlier (*see pages 121–26*). Abdominal breathing, meditation and yoga are direct forms. Interestingly, praying in any

Eastern or Western religion (using mantras, tantras, chants, rosaries and so on) may also have this effect.

Muscle and joint relaxation

Exercise, yoga, massage, the Alexander Technique, osteopathy and many other treatments all have an impact on muscle and joint suppleness. The effect of tense muscles, whether caused by anxiety, poor posture or neurological disorders, is to disrupt sleep.

Pain control

Not only does pain interfere with sleep, but sleep disruption increases the intensity of pain. Many of the alternative techniques have a positive impact on pain, either by alleviating it or at least minimizing it.

COMPLEMENTARY THERAPIES

Method	Description
Acupuncture and Acupressure	Acupuncture is used for a wide range of problems, including back pain. Needles dating back to around 1,000 BC attest to their antiquity. Acupressure uses pressure instead of needles.
Alexander Technique	The Alexander Technique is an educational therapy aimed at improving physical and mental wellbeing by changes in posture. The hypothesis is that habitual bad coordination may lead to excess tension.
Aromatherapy	The use of fragrant oils has developed from the ancient use of aromatic herbs in Egypt, India, Greece and the Arab world. Traditionally, essential oils have been used as stimulants, relaxants, antiseptics and anti-inflammatories. They can alter mood and relieve stress.
Ayurveda	Ayurveda is an Asian medical system that has its beginnings more than 2,000 years ago. 'Ayurveda' literally means 'the science of longevity'. It is an entire system, using herbal remedies, massage, yoga and meditation.
Bach Flower Remedies	Dr Edward Bach developed a range of flower remedies in the 1930s. Morning Glory (*Ipomoea purpurea*) is the remedy most often used to treat sleeplessness.
Biofeedback	Devices provide feedback on various physiological variables like brainwaves, muscle tension and breathing, enabling the user to learn to voluntarily control them.
Biorhythms	Biorhythms have limited scientific support. They rely on a hypothesis that three cycles – physical, emotional and intellectual – affect well-being. They are quite different to the biological clock rhythms described in this book.
Buteyko Method	A breathing re-conditioning program that treats asthma and other respiratory problems.

▶

COMPLEMENTARY THERAPIES

Method	Description
Chinese Medicine	Acupuncture is used for a wide range of problems, including back pain. A complete health system that looks at the body as a balance between the opposite energies of yin and yang. Traditional Chinese medicine includes herbal treatments for almost all known diseases as well as acupuncture, massage, diet and exercise.
Chiropractic	A treatment with the emphasis on re-aligning and adjusting the spinal vertebrae. Manual treatment of many painful conditions, including back pain, sports injuries and asthma.
Colon Hydrotherapy	An infusion of purified water into the colon is said to cleanse and detoxify the inner body.
Counselling	This includes psychotherapy and hypnotherapy. Used for thought management and anxiety relief.
Feng Shui	Feng shui is said to be the practice of living harmoniously with the energy of the surrounding environment. Sleep along a north-south axis, aligning yourself with the earth's magnetic field. If you were born in autumn or winter, your bed should face south and if you were born in spring or summer, your bed should face north.
Hands-on Healing	Generally, hands-on healing and faith healing propose that the mind guides the body and faith healers empower the mind, allowing it to channel its energy to either improve body function or make the body feel better.
Hellerwork	Founded by Joseph Heller, who works from a centre at Mt Shasta, California. It is based on movement education as well as deep tissue manipulation. Used for muscle and joint relaxation.
Herbal Remedies	It is best to visit a herbalist as herbal medicines have virtually no scientific support. The following are often advocated: • CHAMOMILE (*Chamaemelum nobile*) Chamomile tea is a gentle sedative that can help anxiety and promote restful sleep. Chamomile teabags reduce eye inflammation and refresh tired eyes. • HOPS (*Humulus lupulus*) The flower inflorescence is used extensively for the treatment of sleeplessness, except for anyone suffering from depression. • LAVENDER (*Lavendula officinalis*) Lavender oil is used in aromatherapy for anxiety, insomnia and depression. • PASSION FLOWER (*Passiflora incarnata*) The dried leaves are used for treating intransigent insomnia. • PEPPERMINT (*Mentha piperita*) Peppermint is said to promote relief from symptoms that may interfere with normal sleep. It is used to treat nervousness, insomnia and dizziness. • VALERIAN (*Valeriana officinalis*) Valerian is recognized as a sedative and can be found in conventional medical formularies. Herbalists recommend it for nervousness, anxiety, insomnia, headache and intestinal cramps.

Method	Description
Homeopathy	A complete system of complementary medicine based on the idea that a substance that produces a set of symptoms comparable to those present in a disorder can be used to treat the disorder. The remedies are prepared from extracts of plants, minerals, animal and human secretions and tissues.
Hydrotherapy	This therapy is claimed to stimulate blood circulation, draw out heat and provide support while exercising. It is occasionally used for insomnia.
Hypnotherapy	Ancient Egyptians and Greeks are said to have used healing trances. African and American tribal cultures also use drumming and dancing for hypnotic effects. The healing professions have been using trances to implant suggestions for self-cure since the eighteenth century.
Kinesiology	The study of muscle movement. Used for muscle and joint relaxation.
Light Therapy and Bright Light	Light therapy, as currently used, refers to treatments that increase production of vitamin D, thus aiding absorption of some minerals. Bright light can be used to reset the biological clock.
Mindfulness Meditation	Mindfulness meditation techniques are partly based on Eastern meditative practices and so have a long history. Crudely, it involves 'living in the moment', appreciating one's thoughts, feelings and sensations in a non-judgemental way.
Minerals	Deficiency in these minerals – MAGNESIUM, ZINC, COPPER, IRON and CALCIUM – may affect sleep. Reduce levels of ferritin (which carries iron) can result in Restless Legs (see page 143).
Naturopathy	Naturopathic medicine is a natural approach to health and healing that recognizes the integrity of the whole person. It emphasizes the treatment of disease through the stimulation, enhancement and support of the intrinsic healing capacity of the person.
Osteopathy	This is the treatment of painful joints and soft tissue through muscle relaxation and joint articulation techniques.
Melatonin	Melatonin is a brain hormone that provides information for the brain and body that it is dark. In adults it is secreted regularly during the night. It is available as a health-food supplement in some countries and is banned in others. Its use may be confined to chronobiological disorders and possibly jet lag.
Psychotherapy	Psychotherapy usually refers to psychoanalytic or psychodynamic therapy, but can also refer to other psychological treatments that have not been endorsed by professional associations.
Reiki and Seichem	Reiki and Seichem are complete healing systems claiming to benefit those suffering from stress-related conditions.
Shiatsu	Shiatsu is a Japanese massage technique which literally means finger pressure. It promotes deep relaxation and so can help relieve stress.
Tai Chi	Tai Chi is an ancient Chinese exercise system for body, mind and spirit – a form of 'moving meditation'. Its practice improves health, vitality and well-being.
Yoga	Yoga is an ancient form of exercise. Successful practice of yoga can reduce stress and increase suppleness, both of which can benefit sleep.

Index

(page numbers in *italic* refer to illustrations)

Resources and Acknowledgements

RESOURCES

Additional explanatory support that may be needed as well as useful links will be provided via the website www.neuronic.com/ik20.

The NHS provides helpful information on how to get to sleep via the website link www.nhs.uk/live-well/sleep-and-tiredness/how-to-get-to-sleep/ and on insomnia via the website link www.nhs.uk/conditions/insomnia/.

The National Library of Medicine in the USA is a tremendous resource and can be accessed via the website link www.nlm.nih.gov/portals/public.html.

ACKNOWLEDGEMENTS

It is impossible to have done any work without the support of my wife Hilary (and the implicit support from my children Liam, Kim and Dawn).

This book is a 20-year update of the original *Insomnia Kit* edited by Tessa Monina. I have to thank her and Ian Jackson for getting me into this and for the now defunct Smithy's (King's Cross) for keeping me going! In fact the entire Eddison Books team past and present have been a delight to work with.

It is also impossible not to remember the deceased Emeritus Professor Ian Oswald (Edinburgh) whose book *Sleep* brought me, along with many others, into the area.

The technicians who I've worked with have always needed prowess and expertise to get good-quality recordings. Peter Cresswell (not a sleep technician but a great engineer who developed tools for me that could survive even if they fell out of an aircraft), Bobby James, Jane Jones, Lizzie Hill and Stevie Williams were the leads for the larger teams who I also thank.

Eddison Books Limited
Managing Director Lisa Dyer
Managing Editor Nicolette Kaponis
Editor Hugh Barker
Proofreader Jane Donovan
Indexer Stephen Blake
Designers Brazzle Atkins and Gemma Wilson
Illustrator Steve Rawlings
Production Sarah Rooney